25 Natural Ways to Relieve Back Pain

25 Natural Ways to Relieve Back Pain

A Mind-Body Approach
to Health and Well-Being

Romy Fox

Barnes
& Noble
Books
New York

This edition published by Barnes & Noble, Inc.,
by arrangement with McGraw-Hill Professional,
a division of The McGraw-Hill Companies, Inc.

2005 Barnes & Noble Books

ISBN 0-7607-7249-5

Printed and bound in the United States of America

05 06 07 08 09 M 9 8 7 6 5 4 3 2 1

For Larry,
who's put in too many years of back-breaking work.

Contents

Foreword

Back in the early 1970s when I was an internist making hospital rounds in the mornings, attending to a thriving practice in the afternoons, and parenting my seven children in the evenings, I noticed that my foot was behaving strangely when I walked. I had developed a "foot drop," meaning that my foot wouldn't pick up when I walked. Instead, it dragged with each step. This was troubling because I couldn't figure out what was causing it, but I decided to ignore it.

Then I started experiencing shooting pains in the right side of my lower back. When I finally got around to seeing a doctor, the diagnosis was grim: I had a herniated disk, and the only way to fix it was to undergo back surgery. Back surgery? The idea of a scalpel touching my spine definitely didn't appeal to me. At the time, there was very little to speak of in the way of alternative medicine—it was either drugs or surgery, and I wasn't interested in either one.

So instead I decided to cure myself by taking to my bed for the next three months. Today we know that more than a couple days worth of bed rest is actually detrimental, but at that time it looked like the only reasonable choice. I laid in bed about twenty-three hours a day, getting up only to go to the bathroom, take a shower, and do a few back exercises. And after three months, lo and behold, my back was fine! Today, nearly thirty years later, I walk, jog, go to the gym, sit for hours at daylong conferences, and stand in line at the movies without undue discomfort. Oh, and by the way, I never did have back surgery!

The thing that helped me most, I believe, was the back exercises. Back problems are almost entirely mechanical, and once you strengthen your supporting structures you're halfway home. Standing, sitting, and sleeping properly are also absolutely essential. Thirty years ago when my back went out, the only alternatives I knew about were bed rest and exercise. But today there are numerous alternatives, the best of which are contained in this book. I recommend many (if not all) of them to my patients and have seen some excellent results.

Although some back problems require drugs and/or surgery, you may want to try these natural methods before submitting to more drastic measures. I wish I'd had this book thirty years ago when my back was hurting. I'm sure I would have been up and at 'em a lot sooner.

Arnold Fox, M.D.

Introduction—Oh, My Aching Back!

When I was a kid, I never paid one whit of attention to my back. There was no reason to. I did anything and everything without a twinge of pain—from back bends to walkovers to "cannonball flips," a nifty little pool trick during which I'd jump high off the diving board, curl up in a ball, flip forward, and land flat on my back in the water. Pow! You should have seen the splash!

My mother was the first person to make mention of that part of my anatomy, beginning around the time I was eleven years old. "Your posture is terrible," she'd tell me. "Don't sway your back—it makes your stomach stick out," as she simultaneously patted my belly and my rear end, trying to get me to tuck both of them in. She was right; I had that typical lousy posture that you see a lot in little kids, and in some that aren't so little: head jutting forward, shoulders rounded, "wing bones" in my upper back sticking out, lower spine as curved as the letter *C,* gut and rear end in a tug-of-war to see which one could protrude the farthest, and knees locked resolutely back in an effort to support the whole mess.

Mom came up with what she thought was the perfect remedy—ballet class. Ugh! All that stretching and pliéing and jumping around. And I guess she never took a good look at the way ballet dancers stand, or she would have whisked me out of the ballet studio immediately. Ballet dancers in repose stick out their rear ends farther than anybody and are championship knee-lockers! The only difference between them and me, I decided, was that they walked with their feet turned out like ducks. I was more than happy to quit those sweaty little torture sessions before the year was out.

Skip ahead now to me as a twenty-seven-year-old woman, living in my own apartment and vigorously pursuing the (overrated) joys of single life. I wasn't much of an exerciser in those days; maybe twice a month I'd drag myself to the gym. On one particularly fun-filled Saturday morning, as I was making the bed and contemplating (just *contemplating*) a fast twenty minutes on the exercise bike, I leaned forward to arrange the pillows. Suddenly, a pain like I couldn't believe shot through my back, leaving me almost breathless from the shock. *What the heck was that?* When I tried to straighten up, it felt like some demon had permanently locked its jaws on the muscles of my right lower back. Yowling in pain, I grabbed my back and latched on to anything available that would support my weight. Then, assuming the hunched-over posture of my eighty-five-year-old Grandpa Ostrom (who had thrashed his back along with the wheat during harvest season some forty years ago), I staggered to my living room and collapsed, face-first, on the couch. All I could think was, "I'm way too young for this!"

After about a half hour of lying there afraid to move a muscle, I called my friend Rona, who graciously made an appointment for me with her chiropractor, came by to ease me off the couch and into her car (a much more lengthy and complicated process than it sounds), and whisked me off to see the doctor.

So there you have it in a nutshell—my first back attack. I'd love to tell you that it was a fluke and I've never had another, but the truth is there have been too many to count. The good part is that after some twenty years of trying anything and everything to fix my aching back, I consider myself something of a back pain relief expert. That's why I wrote this book, in hopes that (as my mother used to say) "you shouldn't have to go through what I've gone through!"

WHAT'S MAKING YOUR BACK HURT?

A whopping 90 percent of us suffer from significant back pain at some time during our adult lives. That means the odds of experiencing stabbing, shooting, aching, throbbing pain in your spine and surrounding tissues are pretty darn good. And it often doesn't stop there. Back pain can radiate to other parts of the body, cause numbness in the legs, make it difficult to sleep, and trigger anxiety and depression.

Most back pain centers in the lower back (the lumbar region). That's because this area provides you with the bulk of the muscle power you need to lift, stand, and walk, as well as the ability to twist, turn, and bend. A complex structure of bones, cartilage, nerves, joints, muscles, and ligaments, your lower back plays an important part in just about all activities of daily living. That's why it's so devastating when your back is injured; suddenly, it seems like your entire life comes to a screeching halt.

Despite the fact that back pain is so common, its cause is often as mysterious and elusive as a rare butterfly. To make matters even more frustrating, it's often due to a combination of factors. That makes it tough to deal with. It's like an army trying to destroy an enemy without being able to pinpoint its location. Luckily, experts have narrowed down the causes of back pain to five main categories: strains and sprains, disk problems, joint degeneration, osteoporosis, and disease or structural problems. Once you and your doctor have figured out which is most likely to be tormenting you, you can plan your counterattack accordingly.

Strains and Sprains

We've all heard about "weekend warriors" who sit at their computers, in their cars, or in front of the TV six days a week, then on Saturday they suddenly decide to jog five miles, put in a new toilet, and plant a small grove of trees in the backyard. Not surprisingly, on Sunday they're flat on their backs in bed, unable to move or do anything else other than count the flyspecks on the ceiling. That's because they've strained or sprained (overused or even torn) one or more of the muscles, ligaments, and/or tendons in their back. Why did this happen? Two things are usually to blame: poor physical fitness and poor posture.

Disk Problems

"Disks" are the spongy cartilage cushions between the bones (vertebrae) in our spines. They are great shock absorbers and keep the vertebrae from rubbing against each other and wearing each other away. But as we age, our disks begin to get thinner and drier and may even develop small cracks. The vertebrae become more tightly packed together (this is why older people get shorter) and irritate the nerves branching out from the spinal cord and passing through spaces between the vertebrae.

To make matters worse, disks can be injured. My brother-in-law, Larry, is a self-employed building contractor who does everything from roofing houses to remodeling kitchens. One day he took a sledgehammer to a heavy, built-in enamel bathtub, intending to break it into pieces small enough to pull out by hand. But while prying out a piece that was particularly difficult to budge, his back gave way and Larry, not the bathtub, had to be carried out. It turns out that all that stress to his back had caused a "disk protrusion" (a bulging disk). A disk in his lower back had been squashed and was now protruding from its usual place, sort of like a water balloon pressed between two bookends. I guess he was lucky. Sometimes a disk can actually rupture or burst under the pressure. (They call this a "disk extrusion," a "herniated disk," or a "slipped disk.") But whether ruptured or squashed, it's bad news. The injured disk irritates nearby nerves, causing pain to radiate up the spine or down the leg, depending on the nerves involved. In Larry's case, the leg pain was much more agonizing than the back pain since his bulging disk irritated the sciatic nerve, which runs from the lower back, through the buttocks, and down the back of the thigh.

Disks tend to be problem areas for a lot of people—sometimes due to normal aging processes, sometimes due to injury.

Joint Degeneration

The joints of the spine can also start to fall apart as we age. When arthritis settles into the spine, it causes the thinning, drying, and cracking of the disks, with added concerns: stiffness, inflammation, and nerve irritation. And if those thinned-out disks should wear through, the vertebrae will start grinding against each other, causing bony "spurs" or little lumps of bone to form on bone ends to compensate for what's been worn away. Unfortunately, that just makes the bone surfaces rougher and more likely to cause irritation. So it becomes a vicious circle—the wearing away of the bone causes pain and irritation, spurring the body to produce more bone, which makes a rougher surface that causes greater pain and irritation. It's a no-win situation.

Another problem related to joint degeneration is *facet syndrome.* The joints between two vertebrae, called facet joints or gliding joints, allow the vertebrae to move without losing alignment. In facet syndrome, a facet joint becomes inflamed and can cause pain that travels though the nerves and ends up someplace else. So you may feel pain in your thigh, for example, when the inflammation is actually in your back.

While degenerative joint changes are often thought of as "normal" signs of aging, they definitely make back pain and back injury much more likely with age. Oh, the joys of getting older!

Osteoporosis

Bones tend to get thinner, weaker, and more porous as we age, but the process is speeded up in those who develop osteoporosis. This disease is seen a lot in postmenopausal women, people who have been confined to bed for long periods of time and those with a long history of steroid use. Bone tissue is lost at a much faster rate than normal, and the resulting fragile bones are very easily fractured. Osteoporosis of the spine causes back pain and loss of height. In its later stages, the spine can become so weak that it bows under the pressure of holding up the head (causing a "dowager's hump").

Disease or Structural Problems

Sometimes (luckily not often) back pain can be caused by medical conditions such as spinal infections, kidney disease, or cancer. It may also be triggered by deformities of the spine or structural defects such as scoliosis (the spine curves sideways like the letter *S*), lordosis (excessive swayback), or kyphosis (abnormal curve in the upper back).

WHEN SHOULD YOU SEE A DOCTOR?

If your back pain is acute—if it hurts like heck but the pain is generally short lived and you know what caused it (for example, an injury or overdoing it)—you might just want to soldier on without professional help. Of course, you should only do this after seeing your physician to make sure that it's nothing serious and does not require medical care. But if it's chronic—if it goes on indefinitely and doesn't seem to be a response to something definite like an injury—

you will certainly want to see a doctor. A chronically aching back can be a sign of something serious and, at the very least, will put a damper on practically everything you do.

HOW DOES THE DOCTOR DIAGNOSE BACK PAIN?

Your initial visit to the doctor (whether you see a general practitioner, an osteopath, a chiropractor, a sports medicine specialist, or whomever) will probably include the following:

- *An interview,* during which you'll be asked about the intensity and duration of your pain and what seemed to bring it on (for example, an accident, overdoing it, and so on).
- *An examination* of your spine and legs to rule out any serious conditions, such as tumors, infections, or nerve problems that might be causing your pain.
- *Tests,* such as a spinal X ray to look for evidence of arthritis or bone disease, a CT scan or an MRI to look for soft tissue damage, an EMG (electromyography) to look for nerve or muscle damage, or a bone scan to rule out osteoporosis.
- *An attempt to categorize the cause of your back pain.* Putting a name (strain, osteoporosis, and so on) to the problem should at least give you and your doctor a place to begin. But be aware that it's entirely possible for your test results to look normal while your back pain lingers on. Back pain can be extremely difficult to diagnose correctly. In fact, you may never find out what's causing your problem.

Well, that's cheery news, isn't it? On the bright side, most back pain isn't serious and usually disappears within a few weeks at most, whether or not you seek medical attention. But since a few weeks with an aching back can feel like a few *years,* I've got a few suggestions to help you make it through the tough recovery period.

GETTING THROUGH IT—THE FIRST FEW DAYS OF A BACK ATTACK

Back in the 1950s, a family friend named Bob ruptured a disk and suddenly found himself facing surgery. But Bob believed in helping the body heal itself instead of leaping into drug therapy or surgery. He refused the knife and, instead, crawled into bed and stayed there *six solid months,* insisting that rest would cure his ills. Believe it or not, he's had very little trouble with his back since.

In spite of Bob's success, long periods of bed rest are not the recommended therapy for most back problems. In fact, prolonged bed rest actually works against back health. First, too much lying around causes your muscles to atrophy, or get flabby and weak—exactly what you don't want. Second, most people won't rest their backs by lying flat for days on end; instead, they'll prop themselves up on pillows to read or watch TV, assuming some very stressful postures that can do more harm than good. If you absolutely must lie down for a couple of days, make sure it's just that—a couple of days—and that you either lie on your side or on your back with a few pillows under your knees (to help keep the spine straight).

If possible, try to stretch your back a little by lying flat on your back with your knees bent, then grab one of your bent legs and slowly try to bring it to your chest. Hold for a few counts, then slowly bring it down and repeat on the other side. If that goes okay, you might try to bring both knees toward your chest, hold for a few counts, then release.

As soon as you can, get up and walk around, at least a little, and try to resume your normal activities. But be careful. Twisting, bending, and reaching should be kept to an absolute minimum.

When you're suffering from major back pain, just getting into and out of bed and changing positions can be major accomplishments. There are three essential "survival moves" to help you navigate that dangerous territory: the log roll, the sit-up, and the stand-up.

- *The Log Roll*—Obviously, you can't just heave your body from one side to the other in bed, the way you've done all your life. Instead, try this: Lie on your back, bend your knees, and slowly bring them up to your chest. If you can, put a pillow between your knees to keep them from falling to one side and twisting your spine. This keeps your legs aligned with your hip sockets and allows your back to stay in a straight line. Grab your shins with your hands, hold tight, and roll to the side. Your back should remain straight and untwisted this way. Use this same procedure to roll from your side to your back, then over to the other side.
- *The Sit-Up*—It's very important that you go from lying down to sitting up the correct way, or you might damage your back further. Lying on your side, facing the outside edge of the bed, inch your way to the edge. (You might try the log roll if you're pretty far from the edge.) Keeping your legs together, drop your feet and legs off the edge of the bed and lower your feet to the floor. At the same time, push your upper body up off the mattress using the forearm of the arm that's under your body and the palm of the other hand. Your legs will act as a counterweight for your upper body and will help swing you into a sitting position without putting much stress on your back.
- *The Stand-Up*—Once you're sitting up, inch your rear end to the edge of the bed and place your feet firmly on the floor. Tilt your body slightly forward, use your hands to push off (if need be), and stand up. Now that you're on your feet, try walking around a little. You might be surprised at how much better you feel in an upright position!

HOW TO USE THIS BOOK

After your initial examination, the first thing most doctors will want to do for your back pain is write a prescription for pain medication. Now, if you're like me, the thought of taking pain pills is enough to give you a nervous tic; all those horror stories about addiction, grinding stomach ulcers, and feeling "whacked out" in the middle of the day! And if you should visit an orthopedic surgeon, well, don't be surprised if surgery suddenly appears on the treatment menu.

I wrote this book for those of you who want to avoid medication and/or surgery, if at all possible. I believe in the inherent wisdom of the body—that it can and usually will heal itself if treated properly and nudged in the right direction. Of course, medication and/or surgery may be necessary to treat certain serious back problems, but in most cases the more natural, noninvasive approaches can work just as well—and maybe even better.

You can think of this book as a sort of "cookbook" that contains twenty-five of my favorite "recipes" for easing back pain. But take note: *The first ten chapters are the most important.* That's because back pain is almost always due to mechanical problems: the way you stand, sit, sleep, or lift things; weak or overly tight muscles; too much body weight; using your joints improperly; or wearing high heels. *Until you correct these mechanical problems, your back pain is likely to continue.* So concentrate on chapters one through ten first, then either flip through the rest and zero in on whatever looks appealing or read the whole thing before deciding which ones to try.

Some of these remedies might sound a little wacky, while others are based on good old common sense. Some may work for you, others may not, but if done correctly they won't hurt you. Most of them feel good and some are even fun. Taken together, they make up some of the best advice for back pain relief that you'll get from anybody, no matter how pricey the source. So get cookin'! You've got nothing to lose but that ache in your back!

1

Change the Way You Stand

Back in seventh grade I took a class called "Corrective Gym," designed for those of us who failed the posture tests and those of us whose mothers wrote notes specifically requesting that we be placed in this class. I guess you could say that made me doubly qualified. The first thing the teacher did was to analyze each girl's posture, a process that required stripping down to your underwear and standing patiently while she scrutinized your posture from the front, side, and back.

It must have been a good learning experience because I remember the results of her analysis as clearly as if I'd received them yesterday: forward head, round shoulders, kyphosis (rounding of the upper back), lordosis (swaying of the lower back), hyperextended knees (locked knees), and pronated ankles (ankles and arches that bowed inward toward the center of the body). What a mess! What I didn't know is that my posture (which I hope is now my *former* posture) was fairly typical. Loads of people stand with their heads jutting forward, shoulders rounded, backs swayed, and knees locked. The reason? It's easier, especially if your muscles are weak. It's easier to let your head fall forward and your shoulders droop than it is to hold your head erect and your shoulders back. It's easier to lock your knees, letting your joints bear the brunt of your weight, than it is to keep them slightly bent, which calls your muscles into play. And it's easier to let your back sway than it is to tuck your hips under and pull in your stomach.

Unfortunately, this "easy" posture is also the perfect formula for back trouble because it throws your body out of alignment. The result is increased pressure on the disks of your spine, causing excessive wear-and-tear. Bad posture can also strain the ligaments and muscles of your back and neck, irritate your tissues, and weaken the overall structure of your back. Eventually your spine could become permanently misaligned. Standing, sitting, or even sleeping improperly injures your back a little bit every day. And while you may not feel it right now, poor posture will eventually add up to big trouble.

CHANGING THE WAY YOU STAND

Before you can change your posture, you need to know what's wrong with it! Take a tip from my Corrective Gym teacher and do a little posture analysis. Strip down to your underwear and stand sideways in front of a full-length mirror. Hmmm, not bad, right? Okay, now relax a little and stand the way you really do! Do you have any of the following posture problems?

Head and Neck Angled Forward

Ideally, your head should sit right above the center of your torso and the back of your neck should curve in toward your Adam's apple just slightly. Your ears should be straight above the midline of your shoulders (not jutted forward or pulled back). Your eyes should be level with the horizon with your chin dropped slightly, so it's not quite parallel to the floor.

Shoulders Rounded and Chest "Caved-In"

You might think that "correct" posture involves shoulders that are pinned back like a military man, but actually it's somewhere between the slumped posture and the pinned-back one. When your head is erect, your shoulders should line up with your ears and be pressed slightly downward to lengthen your neck and minimize muscle tension from your neck to your shoulders. Pulling back your round shoulders gives you the added bonus of opening up your chest cavity, making it easier to breathe deeply.

Swayed Lower Back, "Pooched-Out" Stomach

Strange as it may sound, your stomach muscles help support your lower back! If you contract them, contract your rear-end muscles, and tuck your rear end under, you can do a lot to take the strain off your lower back and make your muscles do most of the work (instead of your joints).

Dancers and athletes know that speed, power, and balance all come from your "center," an area just above your belly button. Your center can't be strong unless your stomach and rear-end muscles are "engaged." To learn how to engage these muscles, stand with your back to the wall with your head, upper back, and heels firmly pressed against it. Now, tighten your rear end and scoop it under so that your lower back is almost flat against the wall. Then slide your hand between your back and the wall, palm against the wall. If you have the proper amount of lower back curve, you'll have just enough room to slide your hand back and forth easily, while feeling your back and the wall at the same time. (Here's a tip: Bending your knees slightly will make it easier to flatten your lower back.)

Now that you know how to engage your stomach and rear-end muscles, try doing it on a regular basis, when you're standing or walking around. Not only will it be better for your back, it will make you look better, too!

Knees Locked Back

When you lock your knees, it means you've overstraightened your legs to the point where the backs of your knees are actually curving outward. This places the bulk of your body weight squarely on your knees and your lower back, while the muscles that should be supporting you are slacking off. Locked knees also contribute to that awful swayback, stomach-out position. But by keeping your knees just slightly bent at all times, your weight will be more evenly distributed between your joints, muscles, and other supporting structures.

IT AIN'T EASY, BUT IT'S WORTH IT!

If you're not used to standing in this new, improved way, you'll probably find it tiring, and it's easy to slip back into old bad habits. Just make a mental note to keep correcting yourself every time you notice that you're slumping or swaying. Each time you put your body into a better alignment, you're helping prevent the cumulative damage that can add up to a bad back. And you're strengthening muscles that will do a better job of supporting you in the future.

GIVE YOUR BACK A BREAK—BUT NOT LITERALLY!

If you've got back pain, you know that it's not the moving around that kills you—it's the standing around! Waiting in line at the movies, standing endlessly while listening to a museum docent, or inching along through interminable lines at amusement parks can be torture, not only for your back but also for your legs and feet.

I have a friend whose back really hurts her when she stands. The problem is so bad that she won't go to a movie unless she can walk right in without standing in line, or she'll keep walking to the corner and back while her husband stands in line for her. She also shops during off-hours, so she can breeze right through the checkout stands.

If your back hurts, avoid standing for long periods if you can. When you can't, try these tips:

- *Shift your weight*—Stand with your feet about a foot apart, with knees slightly flexed, and transfer your weight back and forth from one foot to another. This relieves some of the pressure on your back, hips, and knees and keeps the blood from pooling in your legs. Military men forced to stand in formation for long periods are told to raise their heels slowly until they've shifted all their weight to the balls of their feet, then to gradually ease back down to a flat-foot position to keep blood circulating—or else they might faint from lack of blood to the brain! While fainting may be the least of your problems, unrelieved pressure on your joints (especially those in your spine) probably is a problem and should be avoided if possible.
- *Stand with one foot higher than the other*—No, I don't mean balance in a tai chi position! But if you should be standing on the sidewalk near a low wall, for example, resting one foot on that wall while your other foot supports you on the sidewalk will take pressure off your lower vertebrae and give you a nice lower back stretch at the same time.
- *Take a hike*—Have someone come with you to stand in line to buy tickets or the line to get in the movies, museums, and so on. While they're standing in line, you can stroll up and down the block.
- *Take along a portable seat*—My husband and I learned the value of this when we took a trip through New England and toured lots of historic houses, museums, and so on. You know how exhausting it can be to follow a tour guide around and then stand in each place for ten minutes listening to him or her talk. That's when we would each whip out a portable campstool, which is simply a triangle of canvas stretched

> between three lightweight aluminum legs. We'd sit down wherever we happened to be, enjoy the lecture, then fold up the stools, sling them over our shoulders using their handy shoulder straps, and be off. I can't tell you how many times other tourists looked longingly at us in our chairs and said, "You guys are smart. I wish I'd brought something like that." You can get a stool like this for under fifteen dollars at any large sporting goods store.

If all else fails, just sit down. Right there on the ground, have a seat. It may not be classy or terribly comfortable, but it beats that unbearable back pain that can come from too much standing.

2

Change the Way You Sit

The longer you live, the more you begin to realize that it's the little things in life that can make or break you. Tiny grains of sand repeatedly washed ashore can eventually create a beautiful beach. Yet, little termites can undermine the structure of an entire building. The same is true of your back. The little things you do habitually every day can either make your back straighter, stronger, and healthier or pave the way to rack and ruin. And one of the biggest little things is the way you sit.

We've all been sitting around since we were infants. Yet this simple act, done incorrectly day in and day out, can be a major cause of poor body alignment, back injury, and pain. For years my own favorite way of sitting was probably the worst on the planet, at least for the back. With my legs stretched straight, I liked to slide down in my office chair until my upper back was completely supported by the back of the chair and my tailbone rested on the front edge of the seat. Then I'd cross my legs at the ankle, fold my arms, and let my chin rest on my chest. Of course, this offered zero support for my lower back (which was sustaining practically all of my body weight), while my poor neck formed a ninety-degree angle to my spine. I usually watched television in bed in a similar position: lower body flat to the mattress, upper body, neck, and head cranked way up courtesy of several pillows. Is it any wonder that I still have neck problems to this day?

Okay, so that's what you *don't* want to do. But what's the right way to sit? Well, proper sitting, especially at a desk or a computer, involves some muscle power on your part. Sit up straight and let your hip bones (rather than your tailbone) bear the weight of your upper body. Slumping causes undue pressure to the vertebrae in your back, especially those in your lower back (lumbar area) and neck. So scoot your rear end all the way back and let the chair support your lower back, while your muscles support your upper back, neck, and head. (If your chair doesn't have built-in support for your lower back, slip a rolled-up towel or cylinder-shaped pillow between your lower back and the back of the chair to help maintain your back's natural curve.) Feet should be flat on the floor, thighs parallel to the floor. (Think ninety-degree angles formed at the hips, knees, and ankles.)

Your shoulders should be relaxed and pulled back to your body's midline, just as you do when standing with good posture. And your head should be erect, not jutting forward, with eyes focused just slightly lower than straight ahead.

It surprised me to learn that looking down at the desk, the way you do when reading or writing by hand, is really stressful for your neck. I was forever leaning on my elbows, angling my head down into the old chin-to-chest position, my whole back assuming the shape of the letter *C.* I thought I was relaxing my body by propping it up like this, but actually that posture was fatiguing. Now, I use a bookstand or a document holder to keep my reading material at an angle that's not stressful to my neck and back. At first it was tiring to try to sit up all day (and I still slump sometimes), but you get used to it after a while. And it has really helped my neck.

THE DO'S AND DON'TS OF SITTING DOWN AND GETTING UP

While we're on the subject of sitting, did you know there's a good way and a bad way to sit down and get up again? Consider these back-saving guidelines.

Sitting Without Stressing Your Back

Instead of just flopping into a chair, try this:

- Standing straight with your back to the chair, back up until you can feel the edge of the chair seat with one of your legs. Position the other leg slightly forward for balance.
- Maintaining the alignment of your head, neck, and back, contract your stomach muscles and release your hips backward to create a "shelf."
- Bend your knees and, using your stomach muscles, lower yourself into the chair. (Don't lean forward!)

Rising from a Chair Without Wreaking Havoc

To get up, do the opposite:

- Sit up tall and scoot to the edge of the chair.
- Place one foot slightly in front of the other and rise, using your thigh muscles.
- Don't use your hands to press on your thighs or the arms of the chair to help you rise unless absolutely necessary. Let your thighs to do the work, instead of your arms or your back.

Sometimes the simplest actions turn out to be the hardest to accomplish, and I think sitting correctly falls into this category. It's not that hard physically, although you do have to constantly remind yourself not to fall back into old habits. But the effort is worth it. Correct sitting posture is one of the most important habits you can establish to save your back. A good chair will be of immense help in maintaining your new posture, as will stretching breaks every fifteen minutes or so to ease muscle stress and strain (see chapter 4). Just remember: Every time you sit up straight and assume a healthier position, even for a minute, you ward off damage to your back. Like sands through an hourglass, these efforts add up.

3

Sleep Your Way to Back Health

You might think that as far as your back is concerned, once you lie down, the pressure's off. Wrong! You can put tremendous stress and strain on your lower back and neck, in particular, just by using the wrong mattress or pillow or by sleeping in certain postures. Since most back pain is due to excessive strain or tensed-up back muscles (both of which can be caused by bad sleeping habits), it's worthwhile to take a peek into your own boudoir and evaluate what's happening to you on a nightly basis.

THE BAD MATTRESS VERSUS THE GOOD MATTRESS

A bad mattress is either too soft or too hard. If it's too soft, your back sags into the mattress (imagine a hammock), and the muscles supporting your spine tense up, valiantly trying to preserve your spine's natural curvature. After eight hours of this, you can understand why your back might feel achy in the morning—especially if this goes on night after night. On the other hand, if your mattress is too hard, your curvaceous and angular body is forced to conform to a perfectly flat surface (think of sleeping on the ground). This will probably leave you tossing, turning, and twisting yourself into all kinds of contorted positions throughout the night.

A good mattress has a firm inner support, with some nice, resilient cushioning on top. This means there will be some "give" to accommodate the sharp angles of your body (knees, elbows, and so on), but your spine will be supported. One brand of mattress currently on the market has a temperature-sensitive covering that allows your body to "make a mold" of itself as you sleep. Yet there is firm support underneath the covering, so you only sink about a half-inch. The most important thing is to find a mattress that feels comfortable day in and day out, and that may be trickier than it sounds. Just lying on a mattress in the showroom for five minutes is probably not going to tell you much. Before you shop, ask your friends if they are satisfied with the mattresses they're using, and get recommendations from your chiropractor or physical therapist. If possible, spend the night on the mattress in question (in a friend's guest room, for example). It may be time consuming, but it's crucial to the health of your back.

THE PILLOW WARS

I am a veteran of the "pillow wars," which is what I call my nightly struggle to support my head and neck. This is very important, because an unsupported neck at night leads to neck pain the next day, and neck pain invariably spreads down the back. That's not surprising, since pain in one part of the body often makes you hold yourself or move in a funny way, and that can cause problems elsewhere.

I've been fighting with my pillows for years now, trying to get comfortable and stay that way, but several times a night I find myself punching, fluffing, folding, or scrunching them—even tossing them out of bed and replacing them with others. And I'm constantly wandering through the bedding section of department stores looking for the magical pillow that's going to ease my neck strain.

I've always slept with at least two pillows under my head, and for a time I even used three! I have a long neck, and one pillow just doesn't seem to support my head well enough. But once my neck started bothering me a lot, I began to pay regular visits to the chiropractor, and he told me about the cervical support pillow. It's shaped like a cylinder, and you put it under your neck when you lie on your back. Your shoulders and the back of your head should lie flat on the mattress, but the pillow supports the curve in your neck. My neck does feel better when I use it, but I can't sleep that way for very long. And when I turn over on my side, that little pillow just isn't high enough. That's when I throw it aside and reach for my two bigger pillows. But after a while my neck starts to hurt, so I throw these pillows aside and reach for my cylinder. Thus, the pillow wars go on at my house on a nightly basis.

The point of this story is that pillow selection is an extremely personal choice. The important thing is to find a pillow that gives good support to your head and neck and doesn't keep waking you up at night. (I'm still searching.) The good news is that there are endless varieties of pillows available, and one may be perfect for you. The disappointing news is that no one can tell you which one is right for you or even what to look for. But I can tell you this: If you find that your neck hurts while you're lying in bed or when you wake up in the morning, the cervical support pillow is worth a try.

SLEEPING POSTURES

I hate to tell you this, but there is actually a good way and a bad way to sleep. (Is nothing sacred?) And I must confess, I sleep in the bad way, which means that I lie on my stomach. My chiropractor, Dr. Dan, literally shuddered when I told him this, before explaining to me that lying on my stomach increases the sway in my back, putting pressure on the disks in my lower spine. It also makes my stomach muscles sag and places too much torque on my neck, since the torso faces straight forward while the head faces the side. (That's okay for stretching purposes in exercise class, but not for hours while you sleep.) Dr. Dan proceeded to tell me that he figured about 80 percent of his patients had back trouble that was primarily due to sleeping in the wrong position!

Okay, so how should we all be sleeping? Well, you've got two choices: on your back or on your side.

Lying on Your Back

This is actually the least stressful lying-down position for the back, but only if you put a cervical support pillow behind your neck and a small pillow beneath your knees, so they stay slightly bent. That way, your entire spine is aligned properly and is well supported. But if you just lie down with your legs completely straightened, you increase the curve of your lower back, stressing it. And if you put pillows under your head, you crunch the vertebrae in your neck.

Lying on Your Side

This may be the most comfortable position for you, especially if you bend your knees equally, as if in the fetal position, and put a pillow beneath your head and neck. That relieves pressure on your disks. Placing a small pillow between your knees can ensure proper alignment of the hips and lower back and can help you avoid twisting your body as your upper knee falls toward the mattress. You can find pillows that strap to your knees so you're not constantly fussing with yet another pillow during the night. That way you can roll from side to side without any hassle.

Okay, so now you've got two perfectly good sleeping positions to use. What more do you want? Well, if you're like me, you want to sleep on your stomach sometimes, too. Or maybe *want* is the wrong word—I just seem to end up that way, no matter what I do. Well, if you can't break the habit, Dr. Dan says you can put a small pillow (yipes, another pillow!) or a towel under your pelvis. That will raise your hips and help straighten out your lower back. I tried it, and it works—at least for a while, until I kicked the pillow out of bed some time around 2:00 A.M. This morning when I woke up, I found five pillows lying on the floor, and I was lying facedown with my cervical support pillow under my forehead. Not exactly what Dr. Dan would have ordered. Oh, well. The pillow wars continue.

4

Embrace Proper Ergonomics

My back and neck always feel worst when I'm sitting at my desk, especially for long hours. That's because hunching over a computer, while reading or typing, is probably one of the most unnatural things I do on a regular basis. Our bodies were designed for prehistoric activities such as walking, running, hunting, gathering, squatting, huddling together, and cuddling our children—in short, we were designed to be on the move much of the day. Yet most of us sit in one place for eight hours a day, staring at the same object. What cave person could have managed that? I did it for years without a second thought. Then I found out that sitting is more stressful to the back than just about anything you can think of—including standing, lying down, and even lifting!

You might think that when you "take a load off" your feet, you're doing the same for your back, but that's not the case. When you sit, your back muscles have to exert extra effort to keep your spine erect. Just think about the last time you sat on the floor and how tiring it was. After a few minutes, you probably began to slouch and search for a place to prop up some of that upper-body weight. Unfortunately, when your back muscles give way like this, all the weight of your upper body begins to rest on the disks of your lower back, resulting in stress, strain, and (eventually) back pain. And you don't have to be sitting on the floor to do a number on your back. If you're sitting in a chair that doesn't provide good back support, you'll end up slouching, which will throw your center of gravity forward and make your hip bones rotate toward the back. The result: stressed-out back muscles.

Throughout the 1950s and 1960s, as more and more people began working at sedentary jobs, the incidence of back pain started to skyrocket. Enter ergonomics, which literally means "the study of work." Scientists observed people who worked at desk jobs and then came up with a list of recommendations regarding the design and placement of equipment that would fit the body, letting it move with the least amount of stress and strain. Among the most important recommendations were specifications for a chair that would help support the back and encourage good sitting posture.

THE BACK-SAVING DESK CHAIR

It's not enough to buy a chair that matches the decor and swivels well. A good chair should have many benefits. Some of the more important qualities of a good chair follow.

Conform to the Shape of Your Spine

That means the inside of the chair back should curve toward you in the lumbar area, so it can lend support to your lower back. (Without good lumbar support, your lower back muscles will always be in a state of semicontraction, and that's tiring!) The lumbar area should provide enough curve so that there isn't any space between your lower back and the chair, but the curve shouldn't be so excessive that it pushes your stomach out.

Provide Good Support Throughout

Beware of squishy chairs! There was a time when business executives favored big, soft, leather chairs they could sink into. But researchers have found that soft chairs make your back do more work—it has to tighten up to hold up your spine. And tense, tight muscles are more likely to tear. Today's execs are more likely to be found sitting on chairs made of a tough, taut, weblike material stretched over an aluminum frame, with just enough "give" to act as a shock absorber when sitting down or shifting positions. But any material that provides good support plus a little resilience will probably do.

Transfer Your Weight Slightly Toward the Back

The chair seat should shift the majority of your weight back, so that it's supported by your pelvis rather than by your thighs. Sitting forward on your thighs puts too much pressure on them and can be bad for your circulation. It will help if you scoot your rear end all the way back on the chair seat.

Change Height Easily

It's important to be able to adjust the height of your chair so that your thighs form a ninety-degree angle to your trunk, your lower legs form a ninety-degree angle to your thighs, and your feet are firmly planted on the floor. (Think of your feet and thighs as stairs in a staircase.) If the chair is too low, your feet and legs can become cramped. If it's too high, your feet can't help support your weight, so your back muscles tense up. (A footrest may solve the problem if everything else is aligned but your feet aren't quite flat on the floor.) An easily accessible height adjustment lever will also eliminate twisting, turning, and bending over while you search for the right knob!

Have Comfortable, Well-Padded Armrests

The armrests should support your forearms and elbows so they make a ninety-degree angle to your body. This helps ease the strain on the wrists (which helps prevent carpal tunnel syndrome) and takes the strain off your neck. (It takes neck and shoulder muscles to hold your forearms and hands at a lower or higher angle.) Armrest padding will eliminate pressure on your elbow joints and forearm bones.

WONDERFUL WORKSTATIONS

These days we're not just glued to our computers at work or at school; we're also glued to them at home! That means you've got two places that may need ergonomic tune-ups. Make sure that:

- The top of your computer screen is slightly below eye level.
- Your eyes are eighteen to twenty-eight inches from the screen.
- Your chin forms a ninety-degree angle to your spine, and your head is erect as you view the screen. (Use a document holder or a bookstand to elevate your reading material.)
- Your shoulders are relaxed (not hunched).
- Your wrists and forearms are level as you type (you could lay a book on them), with elbows supported by the armrests.
- Your files and supplies are easy to reach.

Finally, take plenty of breaks! Stand up, stretch your back and neck, do some shoulder rolls, and shake out your hands. If possible, take a short walk and do some deep breathing. It's an unnatural world that we live in, but we don't have to let it do unnatural things to our backs.

5

Movement Reeducation

When I was a teenager, I had my appendix removed. And, like anyone else with an injury, I put my body through all kinds of contortions as I tried to avoid stressing the surgical site. I practically did back bends trying to get into and out of a chair without bending at the waist, and I spent several nights sleeping in an easy chair since lying on my side was out of the question. But when I think about the pain involved in recovering from that surgery, I really don't remember much of it centering in my abdomen. It was my back that killed me! Between the weird contortions and the bizarre sleeping positions, my back was a mass of aches for weeks.

Something similar may be happening to you if you're living with chronic pain of any kind. By overcompensating and trying to spare a bum knee or a bad back, you may be walking, sitting, sleeping, or otherwise holding your body in a way that brings on even more pain. Or you may just have some bad habits that pay painful dividends in the form of backaches.

In some of the early chapters of this book, we talked about changing the way you stand, sit, or sleep. This chapter will give you some ideas regarding how to go about making those changes. In short, you may need to take a class that teaches you newer, healthier ways of moving—like the Alexander technique, the Feldenkrais Method, or the Trager approach. All three of these methods are great for teaching you how to correct your posture, how to breathe properly, and how to use your body in more efficient, less stressful ways. You'll also learn how to distribute your weight more evenly and how to move injured or damaged areas with less pain and minimal effort. Body awareness is the key, and the instructor will touch you lightly in certain areas to help you learn but will not actually massage you.

THE ALEXANDER TECHNIQUE

An actor named F. Mathias Alexander developed this method when he decided that a stubborn case of laryngitis was actually caused by improper movement and holding too much tension in his body. Alexander believed that poor posture and moving in stressful ways could also bring on emotional problems, in addition to physical ones. Through movement, verbal instruction, and light touching, the practitioner teaches the students less stressful ways of standing, walking, and sitting and increases body awareness. This is sometimes referred to as the "thinking approach" to movement reeducation.

THE FELDENKRAIS METHOD

When physicist and engineer Moshe Feldenkrais faced surgery to heal an old knee injury, he decided there had to be another way. He also happened to be a martial arts expert, which helped him form his philosophy. Deep breathing, improvement of the self-image, working to increase flexibility, and changing unhealthy movement habits helped him ease his pain and avoid the surgical knife. Those who teach this method focus on increasing the students' body awareness by leading them through a series of easy movements that increase flexibility and range of motion while teaching them how the body moves and how to use it more efficiently. Sometimes the practitioner/teacher may teach these exercises by manually moving the student's body through various movements, while the student lies on a mat. This method is a more physical approach to movement reeducation.

THE TRAGER APPROACH

Milton Trager, M.D., was also a boxer and physical fitness enthusiast who believed that pain and stress begin in the mind but can be eased by the manipulation of the body, which can change negative mental and physical habits. The Trager approach is the most intuitive of the three movement reeducation methods. As the practitioner manipulates your body, rocking it, stretching it, and taking your joints through their full range of motion, you relax and become more aware of the link between body and mind. The movements are experienced on a conscious and an unconscious level, and movement becomes associated with pleasure and relaxation rather than with pain.

Since so many of us have back pain that's at least partially due to faulty use of our bodies, it seems logical to take a little time to learn how to use our bodies correctly. Just becoming aware of some of your bad habits sets you on the road toward improvement. But if you don't know what you're doing wrong, how can you possibly make positive changes?

FINDING A PRACTITIONER

If you want to find out more about any of these techniques or find a qualified practitioner, contact: The American Society for the Alexander Technique, 401 East Market Street, Charlottesville, VA 22902; phone: 1-800-473-0620; Web site: www.alexandertech.org;

or The Feldenkrais Guild of North America (FGNA), 524 Ellsworth Street SW, Albany, OR 97321-0143; phone: 1-800-775-2118; Web site: www.feldenkrais.com; or The Trager Institute, 21 Locust Avenue, Mill Valley, CA 94941-2806; phone: (415) 388-2688; Web site: www.trager.com.

6

Use Proper Lifting Techniques

My sister Stephanie traces the origins of her lower back pain to the day she leaned over to pick up her three-year-old daughter and broke just about every rule in the book of safe and healthful lifting. Her feet were close together, she bent from the waist while keeping her knees straight, she had to reach out to get the little one since she was about two feet away, and she relied on her arms and shoulders to do all the work. Not surprisingly, she threw out her back, and it's been very touchy ever since.

Using the correct lifting techniques is important for everybody, but it can really be crucial if you've got back problems. Any time you pick up a load, even a light one, you put stress on your back, especially on your lower spine. And when you think about the number of times that we all bend over and pick up things every day, you'll realize that doing it the wrong way can add up to major back stress over time. Add this to an already weakened back and you've got a recipe for disaster. With so many of us on the brink of a "back attack," it's worthwhile to review the rules of proper lifting, especially since you may not know all of them.

THE RULES FOR PROPER LIFTING

Stand with Your Feet Apart

For maximum leverage and balance, your feet should be about shoulder's width apart. Any closer than that and you'll tend to curve your back when you lift, to maintain your balance. This forces your back to bear the brunt of the weight.

Bring the Load Close to Your Body Before Lifting It

If you have to reach out to grab hold of the load, your arms, shoulders, and (mostly) your back will take on most of the stress. The rule of thumb is the farther away the load is, the more strain it will place on your lower back. Kick, shove, or otherwise move that load to a convenient position for lifting—or walk right up to it yourself, if you can. Don't lift objects crammed into areas that require you to reach for them first!

Bend Your Knees to Reach for the Load, Instead of Bending Over

Keep your back and neck in a straight line with your head erect as you bend your knees and ease toward the underside of the load. Your chest should pitch forward, and your rear end should pitch backward. This squatting stance will put the bulk of the stress of lifting on your legs, rather than on your back.

Slide Both Hands Under the Load

Always use two hands for lifting. Don't try to lift with just one hand, even if it's a light load, because the imbalance can injure your back muscles or upset the alignment of your spine. Make sure you position your hands well under the middle of the load so it will be balanced, and keep the object close to your body. Arms should be straight and elbows and forearms should make contact with the insides of your thighs as you lift.

Use Your Legs to Do the Lifting

Once you've got a good grasp on the load, begin to straighten your legs, keeping your back straight at all times, and rise to a standing position. Do this at a moderate speed—don't jerk up or struggle up too slowly. Jerking and struggling put extra stress on the back.

Reverse the Process When Setting Down the Object

Use your legs to do the work, bending your knees as you ease the load down. Keep the object close to your body, with elbows and forearms touching the insides of your thighs. Keep your back and neck straight; don't bend from the waist.

Stop If You Feel Pain!

Pain is a signal from your body telling you that you're damaging tissue. You shouldn't feel any pain while lifting (muscle exertion isn't the same thing as pain), but if you do, stop immediately. You're doing too much. Find a different way to accomplish your goal, like sliding the load across the floor, using a dolly, or hiring somebody to do it for you. In general, women shouldn't try to lift loads more than about thirty-five pounds, and men should stay away from loads greater than fifty to sixty pounds. But these are just rough estimates—your maximum lifting weight may be much less. Listen to your body.

SMART STRATEGIES FOR MOVING HEAVY LOADS

In addition to the rules for lifting heavy objects, there are some general guidelines for lifting and/or transporting loads.

Push Instead of Pull

It's a lot less stressful to your back to push a load than it is to pull it, so get behind the object whenever possible. (Remember this the next time you're hauling the trash cans out to the curb).

Don't Twist While Lifting

To protect your back, always face straight forward when lifting. If you really want to do a number on your back, just twist to the side before lifting a heavy object. If the object is heavy enough, you're almost guaranteed a strained ligament or herniated disk.

Don't Lift an Object Any Higher Than Your Waist

Hoisting a load above waist-level puts tremendous strain on your lower back and makes you much more likely to sustain a back injury. Trying to put a heavy box up on a shelf is not a back-friendly idea!

Balance the Load

I'm the kind of person who carries three bags of groceries with my right arm so that my left hand will be free to hold my keys. I've also used shoulder purses consistently since eighth grade. Then one day, as I walked down a very narrow aisle in a bookstore with my purse draped over my shoulder as usual, I twisted slightly to the left and (choing!) a muscle in my back went into a spasm. All it took was years of unnatural stress (the purse) plus a slight twist and I had a back attack that lasted for a good week.

I still carry a shoulder purse, but I've lightened its load considerably (just a wallet, brush, and lipstick!), and I make a point of switching it from one shoulder to the next several times during the day. I've also gotten into the habit of carrying grocery bags of roughly equivalent weight in each arm and setting them down at the door while I rummage for my keys. When I buy big 2½-gallon bottles of water (the kind with the handle), I make like the sorcerer's apprentice and carry one in each hand. No unbalanced loads for me. I'm sure that my back appreciates it.

Think Twice Before You Lift

I'm convinced that most back injuries related to lifting are the result of impulsiveness. It's not the well-planned but difficult task like hauling the refrigerator downstairs two flights to the basement or getting the couch through the front door and out to the moving van. It's moving that box of books you've been tripping over for weeks or pulling that carton of picture albums off the top shelf in the closet. You want the job done now, and you're going to get it done come hell or high water! So you go for it—and boy, are you sorry that you did.

All these steps may sound like a lot to remember and go through. I know, I know, plenty of times it's easier to just bend over and yank the box up or reach way out in order to lift something. And when you're digging around in a messy garage or closet, it's hard to use proper form. But if you've got a troublesome back, you can't afford to be careless. Don't subject your back to unnecessary strain—for any reason. And don't think that everything will be fine if you're only lifting light loads. My husband throws his back out at least once a year just by bending over to pick up his shoes or by reaching across the coffee table for his keys.

Plan ahead, think about how you're going to execute the lift, and get help unless you're absolutely sure you can handle it.

7

Get in Shape!

With all the sitting we do, our back muscles have turned into something akin to wet noodles. Think about how little exercise your back gets in a day. If you're like most people, you rarely rely on your back muscles to hold you up completely. When you're sitting down, the back of your seat or chair usually does most of the work of supporting your lower body. When sitting at a desk or table, you can either rely on the back of your chair to support you or you can prop yourself up with your elbows or forearms. The great American pastime of watching TV is often done while lying on the couch or in bed. In fact, chances are you almost always rely on something else to do your back's work for you, except maybe when you're sitting in the stands at your kid's Little League game. And then what do you do? Well, if you're like me, you slump forward and hold your chin in your hands. The result? A weak, underexercised back that's likely to give out when you try to lift something heavy or do some good old-fashioned manual labor.

There's only one solution: *You have to exercise.* You can do a lot to minimize your back pain by doing certain exercises that help strengthen the muscles not only in your back but also in your stomach, hips, and thighs (which help to support the back and/or absorb some of the strain of movement).

I can almost hear the groans arising from couches all over America! But you can do it, and it doesn't have to be drudgery. I know what I'm talking about because, believe it or not, I went back to dance class at the age of thirty-two in order to strengthen my back. No, not the dreaded ballet of my youth (at my age I was not about to tackle pirouettes or the splits!), but a nice lyrical jazz class that had some balletlike moves plus a little funk. It's really fun. And the best part is that dance helped strengthen my back. I have far fewer problems with it than I used to.

But you don't have to put on a pair of tap shoes in order to strengthen your back (or the rest of your body). Following any good exercise program can do the trick; the hard part is finding something that you'll actually do. The possibilities are endless—you can swim, walk, cycle, do Pilates, dance (yes, even ballroom dancing counts), play sports, jog—whatever floats your boat. The best is a combination of several types of exercise so you don't overstress one area while ignoring another. Just make sure you pick the kinds of exercises that you really like so you'll have a good chance of doing them regularly.

A good exercise program includes a short warm-up, some kind of aerobic exercise, strengthening exercises, and a certain amount of stretching to release tension and increase your flexibility.

The warm-up is easy: just do some brisk walking, light jogging in place (if you can manage it), some moderately paced cycling, or anything else that will get your blood going. It should only take about ten minutes before you start to break a sweat. Then you can move into the next phase of exercise with muscles that are primed to do a little work.

During the "work" phase of your exercise routine, alternate between aerobic exercise one day and strengthening exercise the next day. Aerobic exercises are any kind of movement that makes your heart beat faster and your breath come harder (like fast walking, jogging, swimming, or bike riding). Aerobic exercises should be done three times a week for at least twenty minutes per session. That means you need to take a fast-paced twenty-minute walk, swim, or bike ride (no coasting!) just about every other day.

Strengthening exercises are those that help build muscle power and increase stamina. They usually involve the use of resistance—your muscles pulling or pushing against some kind of weight. That weight may be hand-held barbells, exercise machines that have weights attached to pulleys, or just the weight of your own body working against the force of gravity. (A word to the wise: Weight lifting can put a great deal of stress on your lower back, so keep your weights light and get an expert to show you correct techniques.) Like aerobic exercises, strengthening exercises should be done three times a week, for at least fifteen minutes per session. But don't try to do both aerobic and strengthening exercises at the same time—it could be too much. Instead, do aerobic exercises, say, on Monday, Wednesday, and Friday and save your strengthening exercises for Tuesday, Thursday, and Saturday. (You can take Sunday off!)

I'm going to leave it up to you to figure out which aerobic exercises to do, but I can offer some help with the strengthening ones. My dance teacher insists that a straight, strong back is the basis of good health, so we do a lot of great back-strengthening exercises in dance class. (And I've had far fewer problems with my back since I started doing them.) So even if dance isn't your thing, check out these exercises and try adding a few to your strengthening routine. They just might do your back a world of good.

STRENGTHENING EXERCISES

Wall Slide

Objective: To strengthen the back, thigh, and calf muscles

Stand with your back against a wall, feet slightly away from the wall and about eighteen inches apart. Contract your buttocks muscles so that your lower back is flat. Bend your knees and slowly slide your back down the wall until your thighs make a right angle to your back. Hold for five counts, then slowly slide back up the wall. Repeat this five times. (Tip: If this is difficult, you can press your arms against the wall behind you, palms flat, to help you balance. Otherwise, put your hands on your hips.)

Leg Lift

Objective: To strengthen the stomach muscles and stretch the lower back and back of the thigh

Lie flat on your back on an exercise mat, with your arms at your sides, your left knee bent and your right leg straight. Keeping your right leg straight, raise it as high as you can (without lifting your hip off the floor) and hold it at the maximum position for a count of five. Then slowly lower it to the floor. Repeat five times with the right; then bend the right knee, straighten the left leg, and do five leg lifts with the left.

Partial Sit-Up

Objective: To strengthen the stomach muscles

Lie on your back with your knees bent, hands behind your head, and fingertips touching your head lightly. Contract your stomach muscles and raise your head, neck, and shoulders off the mat, trying to keep your head and neck in line with your spine. (Tip: Keep your eyes on the ceiling throughout the exercises and don't bend your neck.) When your shoulders have cleared the floor, you've gone high enough; return your head, neck, and shoulders to the mat. Repeat ten times.

Backward Leg Raises

Objective: To strengthen the lower back and back of the thigh

Lie on your stomach on an exercise mat with your legs straight and together and your arms at your sides. Without lifting your pelvic bones off the mat, tighten your buttocks muscles and lift your right leg off the mat as high as possible. (Don't bend your knee!) Hold for a count of five; then repeat with the other leg. Do five repetitions on each side.

Pelvic Lift

Objective: To strengthen the buttocks muscles

Lie on your back with your knees bent, feet about eighteen inches apart, soles flat on the floor, and arms by your sides. Tighten your buttocks muscles and slowly raise your pelvis off the mat until your spine forms a straight line from your neck to your knees. (Tip: Don't arch your lower back or let your stomach protrude.) Hold that position for five counts, then slowly release, allowing one vertebra at a time to make contact with the mat, beginning with your shoulder area and ending with your tailbone. Repeat this exercise five times.

Backward Leg Push

Objective: To strengthen the back of the thigh and buttocks muscles

Assume a hands-and-knees position on an exercise mat. Bend your right knee and bring it toward your chest, then straighten your leg out behind you, while flexing your foot. (Your leg should be in line with your spine, parallel to the floor.) Keeping your leg straight, raise it just a quarter of an inch, then another quarter of an inch, and a third quarter of an inch. Bend your knee and bring it back to your chest, then place your knee and lower leg back on the mat. Repeat with the other leg. Do this five times on each side.

Back Strengthener

Objective: To strengthen and stretch out the back

Stand with your feet shoulder's width apart. With your knees slightly bent, bend forward at the waist, keeping your back as flat as possible. Raise your arms above your head so that they line up with your back. (Ideally, your arms and back will make a right angle to your legs, and your face will be parallel to the floor.) Now bend your knees a little more, then straighten them a little (don't straighten them all the way). Bend and slightly straighten your knees five times while keeping your arms above your head. Then, drop your arms and bend forward, curving your back and letting your upper body hang. Slowly roll up to a count of eight. Repeat three times.

WHAT'S HOT, WHAT'S NOT

Walking, swimming, cycling, rowing, and jogging are usually helpful because they're good for muscle strength and flexibility and can help reduce back stress. But exercises that involve twisting, lifting, or bodily contact, such as bowling, golf, racquetball, tennis, football, baseball, and basketball can put you at risk for back injury. No matter what kind of exercise you decide to do, it's important that you see your doctor to find out what's appropriate for your condition. You certainly don't want to make things worse.

8

Stretch Away the Pain

My friend Bruce really messed up his back a few years ago when he fell through the trap door of his attic and landed on a ladder, *back first!* Luckily nothing was broken, but it took him a long time to recover, and he continues to have back problems to this day. When I asked him recently about his back pain, he said, "You know, as long as I do my stretching, it's okay. But once I slack off, forget it."

I couldn't agree more. I've found that if I don't do at least a few back stretches every day, my back locks up so tightly that I look like Frankenstein when I walk. And that hurts! But stretching magically pulls most of the tension right out and goes a long way toward relieving my stiffness. One of the smartest decisions I've ever made was to hire a yoga instructor, who taught me some wonderful, therapeutic stretches for the back. After learning the correct techniques and practicing with her for about six months, I joined a yoga class. Today I make a point of going to class twice a week, and the rest of the time I work in at least a few yoga stretches every day, often right before I go to bed. (Yoga is also a good antidote to insomnia.) I truly believe that stretching is the single most important thing I do to maintain the health of my back.

Stretching works on a lot of back problems all at once. Not only does it relieve muscle tension and stiffness, it can also help correct the body's alignment, so you can begin to walk, stand, and move in less stressful, more productive ways. Exercises that stretch your back improve flexibility in the muscles, tendons, and ligaments of your back, shoulders, and legs, so you'll be able to reach and bend more comfortably. And stretching, correctly done, can help prevent future injury to your back. Muscles that are more elastic respond better to sudden movements, twisting, or other stressors to your back muscles. They don't tighten up so quickly and are more likely to "go with the flow."

Stretching is important for everybody, although it may be more important for you, a back pain sufferer. It's a sad fact of life that we all get stiffer and less resilient as we get older. (I'm reminded of my seven-year-old niece who likes to jump up in the air and come crashing down into the splits. Not a trick I'd like to try at my age!) Anybody who wants to maintain his or her current level of flexibility (just maintain it, not improve it), should be doing some stretching every other day. However, those who want to increase their flexibility (and I'm assuming that's you) need to stretch for at least fifteen minutes every single day.

But a word of warning: Don't stretch unsupervised, at least in the beginning. You can do a lot of damage to your already painful back by stretching incorrectly. See a physical therapist, exercise physiologist, or a yoga instructor who's experienced in dealing with back problems for some private sessions before moving into a class. (You can't get the personal attention you need at the outset in a class. Join a class later when you're sure you know what you're doing.) It may be a bit costly, but your back is worth its weight in gold. Treat it that way.

Below I've written a few yoga stretches that are great for the back, just for your information. *Don't try them alone.* Instead, take this book with you to your first exercise session and ask your instructor to teach them to you and make sure you're doing them correctly.

YOGA EXERCISES

Knee-to-Chest with a Twist

Objective: To increase flexibility of the spine

You may remember from the Introduction to this book that when you're having a back attack, it's a good idea to lie on your back with your knees bent, pull them toward your chest, and just hold them there to stretch out the muscles of your lower back. This is a variation on that exercise; one that may be a little too intense when you're in the middle of a back spasm. Try it on one of your better days.

Lie on your back with both legs straight and flat on the floor. Bend your right knee and bring it up to your chest (or as near to your chest as possible). Grab that knee with your left hand and pull it across your body, as if trying to touch it to the floor next to the left side of your body. Your right arm, meanwhile, should be stretched out to the right side, perpendicular to your body. Roll your head to the right and try to look at that right hand. This is a great twisting stretch for your spine. If you can't manage it, just do what you can and hold the position for at least a count of five. Then release and repeat on the other side.

Hamstring Stretch

Objective: To stretch the back of the upper thigh—the hamstrings

Lie on your back with your knees bent, feet flat on the floor, and arms at your side. Grab your right thigh with both hands, fingers wrapped around the back of the thigh, and bring it toward your chest. Keep holding on to your thigh as you straighten your leg. (Lower your leg if necessary in order to straighten it.) Once your knee is straight, hold your leg in that position for a count of five. Return your leg to starting position and repeat with the other leg. Do this stretch at least five times on each side.

The Snake

Objective: To stretch the abdominal muscles, strengthen the upper back and arms, and relax the back

Lie on your stomach, with your elbows bent, palms flat on the floor on either side of your face, and legs slightly apart. Press down with your palms as you slowly push your upper body off the mat, until your arms are completely straight. (Tip: Do not let your head drop either forward or back. Keep your neck in line with your spine.) Hold at this maximum position for five counts, then slowly release and return to lying flat on the mat. Repeat three to five times, depending upon how accustomed your body is to doing this exercise.

The Knot

Objective: To stretch the inner thigh, hip, and lower back

Lie on your back, with your knees bent, and your arms at your sides. Cross your right leg over your left, placing your right foot just beyond your left knee. (Your right knee should be pointing to your right.) Take hold of your left thigh with both hands and gently ease it toward you while keeping your legs in the crossed position. Hold this position for at least five seconds, then gradually release. Repeat on the other side.

Side Stretch

Objective: To stretch the muscles of the side and back

Stand erect, with your feet shoulder's width apart. Put your right hand on your waist, bending your right elbow. Extend your left arm above your head, then bend slowly to the right, keeping your arm above your head. (Tip: To make sure you're bending straight to the side, not forward or backward, imagine there is a wall right in front of your face and right behind your back.) Hold for a count of five, then pull your body up to the standing erect position. Repeat five times, alternating sides.

The Cat

Objective: To stretch the back muscles

Get into a hands-and-knees position on the mat, with your knees slightly apart, neck straight (head should be neither dropped nor arched back), arms straight, and fingers pointed straight ahead. Like a cat, arch your back upward by contracting your abdominal muscles, rolling your shoulders forward, and pulling your chin down until it touches your chest. Hold in this position for a count of five. Then gradually release to your starting position.

From there, gently sway your back, pulling your head toward the back as if you were looking at the ceiling. Don't release your stomach and sink into a huge sway; just a slight one will do. (Too much swaying isn't good for your back.) Hold for a count of five. Then slowly release and return to your original position. Do this arch-sway combination five times.

The Child's Pose

Objective: To stretch the shoulder, back, and thigh muscles

Sit on your mat with your legs and feet folded underneath you, thighs pointing straight ahead. Separate the knees about ten inches, while keeping the heels directly under your hips. Bend forward at the waist until your forehead touches the floor in front of you. Stretch your arms above your head and relax in this position for as long as you like. Then slowly roll up to a sitting position. Repeat, if you desire.

9

Drop Those Excess Pounds

It probably comes as no surprise to you that those extra fifteen pounds you've been carrying around are putting a strain on your lower back. After all, your lower back bears most of the burden of holding up your upper body, and if your upper body weighs a lot, that burden can become hefty. And, as you probably know, excess poundage is bad for any weight-bearing joint. The weight-bearing joints in your lower back are already subject to an awful lot of stress and strain. Add some more weight to the load, and those pounds can really send your back over the edge. It's a well-known fact that most obese people have chronic back problems.

The way your fat is distributed can be even more detrimental to your back. If you carry the extra weight around your middle (particularly in the form of a paunch), your back is at extra risk of injury. That's because abdominal weight is borne primarily by the lumbar (lower back) muscles and ligaments. You can almost hear them groan under the strain of a beer belly, as the back becomes increasingly swayed and the lumbar disks squash together. The same thing happens during the latter stages of pregnancy, when low-back aches and pains due to the extra load "out front" can become tremendous. In both cases, the center of gravity shifts forward, and the lower back must curve even more to support it. On the other hand, if the bulk of your excess weight lies in your hips and legs, it may not make much difference at all to your back.

The relaxed abdominal muscles that usually go along with "paunchiness" can be bad for the back. But toned, tight stomach muscles help maintain body alignment and help take some of the stress off the lower back. Just think of what happens to your back when you "let it all hang out" in front. Instantly, your lower back sways. But when you pull in your stomach muscles, your hips automatically roll under, and your lower back curves less. You can help your back immensely just by losing weight (if you need to) and tightening up your stomach muscles.

If this were a perfect world, I'd now give you a quick and easy way to lose weight and keep it off forever—but, of course, you and I both know better. If you need to lose weight, you've probably already tried a lot of the fast and fancy diet plans currently being touted and found out what I've found out—they don't work. Or they do work, but not for long. So I'm not going to give you any magic eating plan. Instead, I'm going to tell you what I personally have found most helpful in waging war on extra pounds.

I struggled with a weight problem for about ten years. I was lucky enough to be skinny as a child, but that ended at age nineteen when I moved into the dorms at college. There, I started packing on the pounds as I ate my way through three hefty meals a day and plenty of late-night snacks. Then I moved into an apartment with three other girls, and our favorite thing to do was eat globs of peanut butter straight out of the jar, drizzled with honey. Chocolate chip cookie dough was another favorite, as was cream cheese frosting (straight or on graham crackers). Anyway, I wound up weighing between fifteen and twenty pounds more than I should have. Okay, no big deal, you might think. You can drop that pretty easily. The trouble was, I never could. I carried the weight for ten long years and couldn't seem to budge it, no matter what diet I tried.

During those ten years, I came to realize a few things about myself. First, the minute I put myself on a "diet," all I wanted to do was eat. I suddenly got hungry and food-obsessed in a way that I'd never been when I wasn't dieting, even if I was actually consuming more food. Second, diets made me nervous—and when I got nervous, I ate. Third, if the diet said "eat four slices of bread a day," I automatically had to have five. So diets were out, as far as I was concerned. But guess what? I eventually dropped all the weight and I haven't regained it, many years later. So in this chapter, instead of outlining some annoying food-combination method for you or telling you to eat three ounces of fish, half a cup of vegetables, half a cup of rice, and one fruit for lunch, I thought it might be more helpful to give you the skinny on how I, personally, dropped my weight.

ROMY FOX'S RELAXED-BUT-SMART-WAY-TO-SLIM-DOWN-BUT-STAY-SANE DIET

1. If you really want to eat something (say, a hot fudge sundae), go ahead. Just make sure you *really* want it. Otherwise, skip it.
2. When you eat that special something, sit down, eat it slowly, and really savor the flavors. Don't read, watch television, drive your car, or do anything else that will take your mind off the experience.
3. The minute you feel satisfied, stop eating. I've thrown away ice-cream cones half-finished because I suddenly realized that I'd eaten all I wanted. This also holds true for a meal. Tune in to your body, and the second you feel full, stop eating. Put the food away immediately, and don't eat again until you're truly hungry.

4. Remind yourself that *you can always have more later.* This is important; otherwise you start feeling deprived. And when you really do want more, help yourself.
5. *Always* eat breakfast, lunch, and dinner. No skipping for any reason!
6. *Always* eat something when you feel hungry. Your stomach is growling for a reason. Don't let your blood sugar dip too low, or you'll find yourself ready to gobble up an entire box of cookies.
7. Bring snacks with you to work or school. You know you're going to get hungry some time during that long stretch between lunch and dinner. Wrap up some healthy snacks such as carrot sticks, fruit, yogurt, or cereal so you'll have something to munch on instead of the junk in the vending machine. As for convenience, there's no faster fast food than an apple. No standing in line to place your order, no driving through the drive-through. Just reach into your purse or briefcase, take out the apple you put there this morning, and start eating.
8. In general, try to follow the principles of good nutrition. Plan your meals to include plenty of vegetables, legumes, fruits, and whole grains, with smaller amounts of lean meats and dairy products.
9. Use low-fat or nonfat dairy products, margarine, salad dressings, and so on whenever possible.
10. If you must drink soda, learn to drink the diet kind. Why would you want to slurp up 150 calories when you could slurp just 1 calorie?

Most of all, don't compare yourself to others, especially not those ridiculously skinny models in the magazines. And don't fret if you don't weigh what you "should" weigh. This will only upset you, and the "I'm upset" part of the brain is directly connected to the "I've got to stuff myself" part.

10

Dump the High Heels!

Oh ladies, believe me, I know! Nothing in the world can make you look taller, slimmer, or sexier than donning a pair of high heels. Suddenly your legs are two inches longer, your calves take on more shapely lines, and your rear end perches higher on your pelvic bones and acquires an attractive little wiggle when you walk. There's definitely a reason that Miss America contestants parade around in the unlikely combination of heels and a swimsuit.

You're probably well aware of the disastrous effect of high heels on your feet. Anybody who has ever been foolish enough to wear heels while shopping knows all too well about the pain, fatigue, blisters, and sore muscles they can cause. That's because high heels throw your body into a completely unnatural position from the waist down. The entire force of the body's weight is suddenly borne by the ball of the foot as the metatarsal bones are cranked almost to a ninety-degree angle. To add insult to injury, high heels usually have pointed toes that squeeze your toes in toward the middle of your foot, encouraging bunions, corns, and calluses. It's no wonder that 90 percent of today's foot surgeries are performed on women!

But what might surprise you is the effect that high heels have on your back. Because your feet are the foundation of your body, the bizarre alignment created by high heels throws everything above them out of whack. The tendons in your calves contract and shorten, making tendinitis a possibility once you take off your heels and stretch out those muscles. Your knees can become misaligned, causing their cartilage to wear unevenly, leading to osteoarthritis. (Women are twice as likely as men to get osteoarthritis of the knee.) And high heels make your pelvis jut toward the rear, putting stress on the hip joints. All of this leads to the inevitable squeezing together of the vertebrae in the lower back, causing a swayback. This puts a great deal of strain on both the muscles and the disks of the lower back—a major cause of lower back pain.

And the thin, unpadded soles found in most high heels absorb almost none of the impact as your feet strike the ground. The shock waves radiate straight up your legs and settle in your lower back.

So does this mean that you're stuck with a choice of either sensible brown oxfords or the flat, thickly padded sandals that Grandma used to wear? No, although either probably *would* be the best thing for your back, legs, and feet. But let's get real! You like to look a certain way, especially when you dress up, and tennis shoes aren't going to make it with that new satin halter dress you just bought. So here are a few practical guidelines for wearing high heels:

- If you want to wear some kind of heels to work, stick to those no higher than one and a half inches. Pumps should have a square or roundish toe box so your toes aren't squashed. And the more padding they have in the sole, the less impact your back and legs are going to feel.
- Wear flats or tennis shoes whenever you'll be walking any farther than about a block. That means if it's a trek to your car or to your favorite lunchtime hangout on workdays, bring your tennis shoes along and change into them at the appropriate time. It's a hassle, I'll grant you, but your back, legs, and feet will thank you for it.

- Save high heels (taller than one and a half inches) for special occasions only—that means you *won't* be wearing them to work, school, or the mall. But if you happen to be going to a wedding, a formal dinner, or some other dressy affair and want to look smashing, go for it.

So now I'm going to assume you're wearing shoes of the proper height at all times. But it's just as important to wear shoes with the proper fit. Although it might seem obvious to say this, you should only buy shoes that feel good *the very first time you try them on.* This is a foreign idea to most women. We *expect* shoes to hurt when we try them on in the store. "They'll stretch out once I break them in," we tell ourselves. But if you ask the man in your life if he'd buy a pair of shoes that hurt a little bit when he tried them on, he'll tell you, "No way! If the shoes don't feel perfect in the store, I don't buy them." We women are just so used to focusing on the look of the shoes rather than the *feel;* we've brainwashed ourselves into thinking that uncomfortable shoes are okay. From now on, do what the men do: If the shoes don't feel good *right away,* don't pull out your checkbook.

So what should you be looking for in a pair of good, well-fitting shoes (whether high heels or tennies)? Consider the following tips:

- In closed-toe shoes, the area that surrounds your toes (the toe box) should be roomy enough so your toes can wiggle, although your foot shouldn't be able to slide from side to side. The tops of your toes shouldn't rub against the toe box.
- The area that surrounds your heel (the heel counter) should support your heel and keep it straight up while you walk and stand, rather than allowing your heel to slip toward the inside or outside of your shoe. The heel counter should always be made of strong, durable material but shouldn't rub against your heel in any way.

- The insole of your shoe (the inner sole that goes from the heel up to the toe area) should be well padded, especially underneath the heel. This padded area beneath your heel should extend all the way to the edge of the heel counter and should be elevated slightly above the toe area.
- The shoe should provide support for your arch that reflects the natural curve of your arch (or, if you have flat feet, what the natural curve should be). Without arch support, your feet may tend to rock inward toward the inside of your ankles, throwing off your body's alignment.
- The sole of the shoe should be somewhat flexible, bending and straightening along with your foot as you walk (think tennis shoes). Soles that won't bend with your foot can alter the way you walk, and that's bound to affect your body's alignment. You don't want them to be too flexible, though (think flat ballet shoes), because they won't provide adequate support for your arches.

If you do wear shoes with a heel, don't wear them every day. Choose athletic shoes or flats as often as possible to give your feet, legs, and back a break. And keep an eye on how your shoes are wearing—worn-down heels (especially if they're unevenly worn) can make your foot unstable and throw your alignment out of whack. Send them to the shoe repair shop for new heels ASAP.

11

Heat and Chill the Pain Away

So far, all of the remedies I've recommended for back pain are designed to attack the problem at its root. By correcting your posture, using ergonomically correct furniture, doing exercises to strengthen and stretch your back, wearing comfortable and supportive shoes, lifting things properly, and losing excess weight, you can go a long way toward easing back pain today and preventing it from showing up tomorrow. Hot and cold therapies, on the other hand, are designed to make you feel better, but they probably aren't going to correct or prevent any problems. They are strictly "for the moment" remedies.

In general, heat is used to ease muscle stiffness and soreness, while cold is used to help reduce swelling. There's some argument among professionals who treat back problems as to which is better, heat or cold. Some doctors and physical therapists think you should ice your back after a wrenching injury for at least the first forty-eight hours to ease spasms and swelling. But others think you should apply moist heat or lie in a warm bath to help relax the muscles. Still others like the idea of alternating heat and cold. Since the jury is still out on this one, check with your doctor to find out which treatments are appropriate for you. Unless there are signs of inflammation, the doctor will probably tell you to do whatever feels best.

But a word of warning: Heat might make certain conditions worse. Inflammation should always be treated with cold therapies, switching to heat only after the swelling has subsided. Avoid hot baths or whirlpools if you have a fever, a heart condition, or an injury that is bleeding. Don't apply heat if you have an infection. And if pain or inflammation increases after using heat, stop and call your doctor.

HOT THERAPIES

I love heat. It can help relieve pain, relax the muscles, and increase the flow of blood to the injured area, which should help it heal faster. Besides that, it's just a good cozy feeling. And there are lots of soothing, comforting ways to deliver heat to your injured or painful back, including:

- *Hot compresses*—You can buy heat packs containing special chemicals that release heat when the pack is crunched up, or another kind that can be popped into the microwave for a minute before being applied to your back. Or make one yourself: Fill a man's clean sock with uncooked rice, tie it securely, and put it in the microwave for two minutes. Then drape the rice-filled sock over the painful part of your back. The rice will hold the heat for an amazingly long time.
- *Hot-water bottles*—Here's an old-fashioned but great way to deliver heat to your painful area. Wrap the hot-water bottle in a towel to preserve the heat and to keep from burning your skin.
- *Heating pads*—These electrical devices are like mini-electric blankets, complete with dials to control the amount of heat

delivered. If you buy the waterproof version, you can wrap a damp towel around it to provide moist heat.

- *Electric blankets*—Here's a good way to relax your entire body without delivering too much heat to any one spot.
- *Heat lamps*—An infrared light will deliver heat directly to the desired spot.
- *Warm showers*—A steady shower of warm water on your back is very relaxing, especially if you get one of those special showerheads that delivers a machine gun-like massage spray.
- *Warm baths*—The great thing about a warm bath is you can truly relax, since you're lying down. However, lying in the typical tub can crunch your neck vertebrae. Try slipping a waterproof pillow under your upper back to help straighten out your spine.
- *Hot blankets*—Toss a blanket or flannel sheet into the dryer for a few minutes, then spread it over the injured area or use it to cover up your whole body.
- *Whirlpools*—Hop into a whirlpool bath and, if you like, center your painful area right over one of the jets.
- *Ultrasound*—This is a fancier way to produce deep-tissue heat, using high-frequency sound waves to rev up circulation and to relax the muscles in a specific area. Of course, you'll need access to an ultrasound machine, or a visit to your doctor or physical therapist may be in order.

Not only are hot therapies a good way to ease back pain and stiffness due to injuries, they're also a great way to relax the muscles and warm them up before exercising. Try a warm shower or a few minutes in the Jacuzzi before you take your next brisk walk. It will probably make your back feel better and function more effectively. Or how about a warm bath or a hot compress before you do your stretching? I'm betting you'll find it a lot easier to touch your toes!

Too Much of a Good Thing

Of course, anytime you use heat, there's a possibility that you might get burned, if you're not careful. So be sure to protect yourself from skin damage and other problems by following these rules:

- Keep heating pads on low or medium, and make sure bath water doesn't exceed 105° Fahrenheit. (It should feel comfortable on the inside of your elbow.)
- Don't apply heat to any given area more than three times a day or for more than thirty minutes each session.
- Insulate hot compresses or heating pads with towels; don't place them in direct contact with your skin.
- Keep your skin dry and free of creams or lotions (especially deep-heat creams) to prevent allergic reactions or steam burns.
- Check the area every five minutes for reddish-purple skin, blisters, or hives.
- Don't reapply heat until your skin has returned to its normal temperature.

COLD THERAPIES

Cold therapies work mostly by numbing the painful area. Although at first they tend to slow down the flow of blood, eventually the cold helps to increase the circulation. (Once your body gets over the shock, it rises to the occasion and revs up the blood flow.) Cold packs are used to reduce inflammation, ease muscle spasms, and block pain signals. The most obvious way to chill a part of the body is to use ice packs, but you can accomplish the same results in several ways, as follows:

- *Cold packs*—Ice cubes or crushed ice placed in a plastic bag or a hot-water bottle will certainly do the trick, but you can also use commercial cold packs—soft, flexible plastic containers filled with gel. This gel takes a long time to thaw, so you won't have to keep running to the freezer for new supplies. And, unlike ice, it won't drip. You can also try a plastic bag filled with frozen peas, which can mold to your painful area much better than can a bag of ice cubes. Unfortunately, it will drip, so make sure you wrap it snugly in a towel first.

- *Cool compresses*—A cool compress is a less stringent way of easing pain and inflammation. The easiest way to make one is to immerse a washcloth in ice water, wring it out, fold it, and lay it on the affected area.
- *Short, cold baths*—If you're a member of the Polar Bears Club, you might not mind a short plunge into a cold (or cool) bath to help numb the pain and increase circulation.
- *Short, cold showers*—When Prince Charles attended boarding school in Scotland, a cold shower was *de rigueur* every single morning. It certainly must be an invigorating way to start the day!

But Don't Chill Out Too Much!

As with heat, applying cold can damage your skin and other tissues if you do it incorrectly. To avoid frostbite, follow these tips:

- Don't apply cold for longer than twenty minutes.
- When the area becomes numb, discontinue the therapy.
- Check your skin for redness or white areas.
- Don't use cold therapies if you have heart problems, bad circulation, damaged nerves, or decreased sensation.
- If it hurts, stop.

12

Consider Chiropractic

Developed in the late 1800s by Daniel David Palmer, chiropractic is based on the idea that the body can heal itself through the power of the central nervous system. But the nervous system, which is made up of the brain, spinal cord, and the nerves, can be damaged or blocked when misalignments in the spinal vertebrae put pressure on nearby nerves. The tissues or organs served by these "squished" nerves may become diseased or damaged and can no longer function as they should. But manipulating the spine and releasing the pressure on the nerves can eliminate illness and restore health. So, theoretically, the pain in your arm may be due to pressure on a nerve in your back.

Misaligned vertebrae that put pressure on nearby nerves are called *subluxations,* and your chiropractor may try to correct your spine's misalignments in one or more ways. He or she might first use some methods of *spinal manipulative therapy* (SMT), such as massage, acupressure, or other kinds of bodywork to relieve your pain, release stress, and restore function. He or she might also use an *activator,* a tool that looks like a miniature pogo stick with a rubber tip. By applying the activator to certain points on your body and pulling the "trigger," the chiropractor releases a direct, precise force that can help push misaligned vertebrae back into alignment. And then there's the good old trick of "cracking" your neck or back. The chiropractor does this by taking your joint past the point where it wants to go (its passive range of motion) but not farther than it can go anatomically. When this is done, gasses are released within the joint fluid and you hear a "pop" or cracking noise.

To tell you the truth, it took me a long time before I could muster enough courage to visit a chiropractor because I wasn't crazy about the idea of getting my back or neck cracked. So I read about chiropractic a lot before committing myself and found that dangerous complications resulting from neck or back adjustments were extremely rare—maybe fewer than one in a million. The odds were better that I'd hit the jackpot next time I played the dollar slot machines in Vegas. So I figured I was pretty safe.

But I still wasn't really convinced that chiropractic could do anything for my back and neck problems. The fact that more than fifty million Americans swore by their chiropractors and that it was the third largest health care profession in the country didn't really sway me. I wanted to find out exactly what chiropractic could do for me before I handed over my spine for manipulation purposes. So I started reading the results of studies and found that chiropractic manipulation of the lower back really can speed up a person's recovery from acute, uncomplicated lower-back pain (the kind you get when you suddenly throw out your back). Chiropractic can also help relieve pain due to a "slipped disk" or sciatica (pain that radiates from your lower back down through the back of your thigh), and it may also be useful in treating muscle spasms, headaches, shoulder, and knee pain. As for neck pain, chiropractic treatment is every bit as effective, or even more than, traditional medical treatments. (This last one is not too surprising, considering that physicians really don't know what to do for back or neck pain. The standard traditional medical treatment includes a couple of days of bed rest, application of cold or hot packs, mild stretching exercises, and the use of pain relievers as necessary. Chiropractic, on the other hand, attacks the root of the problem.)

So, I decided to bite. I got the name of the chiropractor my best friend uses, a man named Dr. Dan (he uses his first name to keep the formality levels down), and made an appointment.

Dr. Dan and I had our first meeting face-to-face in his office, where we talked about what was hurting me (at the time it was my neck, no surprise), the kind of pain it was (achy, moderate), and how long I'd had it (months, even years). He took an X ray of my neck, then led me to the adjustment room where I lay facedown on a padded table. Dr. Dan felt along my spine, looking for tense muscles, vertebrae that were out of line, inflammation, or anything else that seemed abnormal. Then he used the activator, which gave a tiny, controlled power-punch to various areas along my neck, spine, and even the backs of my legs. It didn't hurt at all. After that, he pressed his thumbs really hard into a spot on either side of my neck and held it for about a minute (although it seemed like an hour), using a technique he called *Trigger Point Therapy.* Now *that* hurt, but when he was through, the muscles in my neck had magically released their tension. My neck hadn't felt so good in ages! And surprise, surprise—no cracking! Dr. Dan said that the activator was so effective that cracking was now an option in most chiropractic treatments, rather than a necessity.

Just to confuse things a bit, there are two types of chiropractors, often called the *straights* and the *mixed.* Straight chiropractors are firm believers in subluxations and spinal manipulation; they focus exclusively on finding and fixing the problems caused by pressure on the spinal nerves. Mixed chiropractors go further, incorporating diet, supplements, and other therapies.

But remember: There are good chiropractors and bad chiropractors, whether straight or mixed. I personally knew one who had an assistant set up the patients and get everything ready for him. Then he came into the examining room, did a quick crunch, crunch, and left. He actually bragged to me that he spent no more than five minutes with each patient! Make sure you find one who spends at least twenty minutes with you each session and who always performs some sort of massage or soft-tissue manipulation before doing the adjustment. (Back-massaging beds, vibrators, or other devices don't count! In general, the more gimmicks and gadgets the chiropractor uses, the faster you should run out the door.) Also, beware of chiropractors who take more than one or two X rays (if that); it's usually not necessary and it's a great way to run up your bill. And watch out for other methods of separating you from your money—like selling you vitamins, food supplements, or health potions. You can purchase these items for less at the health food store, and who needs to endure yet another sales pitch?

Most people who use chiropractic are happy with the results, but if you don't notice a difference after a session or two, hang in there. Sometimes it takes five or six adjustments before it "takes," or perhaps another chiropractor might be a better fit for you. Try someone else before you give up. There's a good chance your persistence will pay off.

FINDING A PRACTITIONER

If you're in the market for a chiropractor, you might begin by asking your doctor, physical therapist, massage therapist, and/or your friends for recommendations. Since chiropractic is so popular these days, you probably won't be at a loss for referrals. If chiropractic is covered by your insurance plan, it makes sense to try someone on their preferred list. You can also contact the American Chiropractic Association, 1701 Clarendon Boulevard, Arlington, VA 22209; phone: 1-800-986-4636; Web site: www.amerchiro.org.

13

Get a Massage

Probably the oldest method of treating back pain is the good old-fashioned massage. Derived from the Arabic word *massa,* which means "to stroke," massage involves the hands-on rubbing, kneading, stroking, and/or application of pressure to the skin and the muscles that lie beneath it. A good massage is an infinitely relaxing and sensuous experience that can help relieve tension, loosen muscles, increase circulation, and calm nerves. It can also help relieve pain by clearing away some of the irritating by-products of muscle metabolism.

Massage produces some wonderful bodywide effects, too. As tension levels decline, the heart rate slows, and overall relaxation greatly increases. There's a marked increase in the level of endorphins, the body's "feel-good" hormones, decreasing pain and producing a wonderful natural "high." (Who needs a glass of wine?)

Massage also helps to melt away mental stress, relieving not just your mind but your body as well. Have you ever noticed that when you're under stress, you're a lot more likely to catch a cold? (I never once made it through final exams without having a runny nose!) That's because stress tends to weaken the immune system. When you're under stress, your body releases powerful chemicals such as cortisol that suppress immune function. But some studies have found that massage may be able to lower cortisol levels, freeing the immune system to do its job.

Massage also promotes circulation of the lymph, the milky white fluid that carries away impurities and waste. Lymph doesn't simply flow along the way blood does, but is propelled along through the system by the squeezing action of muscle contractions. Massage produces this same squeezing effect, so toxins get moving and can be flushed out of the body faster.

There are all kinds of massage, but the most popular form in the United States is Swedish massage, or *effleurage.* The skin and muscles are gently kneaded and stroked, and pressure is exerted on muscles that are tense. Sometimes the therapist may also use tapping or clapping movements. Another common form of massage is *shiatsu* (also known as acupressure), which is used to release energy blockages and restore the flow of the life force *qi.* Many massage therapists do a combination of these two. There are lots of other massage techniques, too, involving deep muscle massage, pressure placed on certain trigger points, the use of wooden rollers or pointers, and manipulation of various joints like the shoulder, and so on. But the general idea remains the same—release muscle tension to promote relaxation.

Before you begin with a new massage therapist, have an in-depth talk about the state of your health, what hurts, what you're looking for in a massage, what you like, what you don't like, and so on. Most therapists can perform several kinds of massage, so ask yours what's available and decide which kind(s) you'd like to try.

Take a warm bath or shower just before your massage to get a jump-start on relaxation. Don't apply any lotion or oil to your skin. Arrive on time so you won't be rushed or stressed. Don't drink alcohol or eat for an hour or two before your session.

I got my first massage about fifteen years ago and would have instantly become an addict except that it's fairly expensive. It did take me a few minutes to get used to the whole process, though—handing over my body to a virtual stranger to be touched, stroked, and manipulated felt a little funny at first. But when I finally let down my guard and decided to trust the therapist, I experienced a deeply relaxed feeling that I hadn't known before.

If you're new to massage and feel awkward about shedding your clothes, then leave some of them on! You can even get massaged while fully clothed, if you like. But it really is best if the massage therapist can work directly on your skin, using oils and lotions that can make his or her hands slide easily over your body. You don't have to worry that you'll be lying on the table, exposed. Every time I've received a massage, I've been completely covered with a flannel sheet, which is rolled back to reveal only the area that the therapist is working on at the moment (like a leg or an arm). Then, as soon as that part is massaged, it is immediately covered up again. Not embarrassing at all!

But speaking of embarrassing, some people do find it awkward to be massaged by a member of the opposite sex—or, in other cases, a member of the same sex. My friend Joan, a lovely sixty-five-year-old woman, received a massage from a young man one time. She tried to relax, but it made her so nervous to be massaged by a man that she clamped her legs tightly together the entire time. I've also known men who insisted that only women could touch them. The point is, you need to figure out in advance if the sex of the therapist is going to be an issue, then make a choice, if necessary. Don't just go along with whoever is available. You need to feel comfortable with and to trust your therapist if you are going to relax fully.

Once you've decided on a therapist and the clothes/no-clothes issue, you'll lie on your stomach on a padded table that's covered with a flannel sheet, and you'll be covered by a flannel sheet as well. The therapist may play soft music and turn the lights down low to promote a relaxed feeling. Once the massage has begun, try to let go as much as possible and allow the therapist to work his or her magic on your body. Breathe deeply and slowly. If you're new to massage, this may be a bit difficult because you aren't quite sure what to expect. But, over time, as you get to know and trust your therapist, you'll probably be able to stop worrying and just enjoy the process. Some people like to talk during the massage; it's a release for them. Others like to be silent and drift into a dreamlike state. Do whatever seems most comfortable to you.

After an hour or so on the table, you should be feeling about as limp and relaxed as a wet noodle. Take a few extra minutes to lie there and regroup before you get up and get dressed. Be sure to treat yourself gently: move slowly, breathe deeply and rhythmically, and try to maintain that wonderfully relaxed state, even as you dress and go out into the world again. If you can avoid it, don't jump immediately into heavy traffic or any other stressful situation. Instead, try to get home and take a nap as soon as possible. And don't forget to drink plenty of water. Drinking extra water will help flush out toxins.

FINDING A PRACTITIONER

You can begin your search for a good massage therapist by asking your physical therapist, chiropractor, or friends for recommendations. You can also contact the American Massage Therapy Association, 820 Davis Street, Suite 100, Evanston, IL 60201; phone: (847) 864-0123; Web site: www.amtamassage.org; or the National Certification Board for Therapeutic Massage and Bodywork, 8301 Greensboro Drive, Suite 300, McLean, VA 22102; phone: 1-800-296-0664; Web site: www.ncbtmb.com.

14

"Pin" and "Press" the Pain Away

When I first heard about the traditional Chinese medical treatment called acupuncture, my reaction was, "Hmm. Interesting, but definitely not for me." The last thing I wanted to do was offer myself as a pincushion. Let someone stick a million needles into me—are you kidding? The way I saw it, needles *caused* pain; they didn't cure it! But my best friend Maggie (another victim of back pain) had gotten such good results from acupuncture, I finally decided to try it.

Guess what? It really doesn't hurt at all. Yes, they do stick needles into your painful area, but they're very thin (hardly thicker than a hair), and in my case they were inserted just below the skin. (I have heard that they can be inserted as far as about an inch, though.) I've had about twenty sessions now, and have sometimes felt the slightest pricking sensation when the needles went in, but after that, nothing. Then, my doctor hooks up the needles to a machine that delivers a very low-level electrical current that you *can* feel, but it's actually kind of pleasant—as if your nerves are getting massaged with a tiny vibrator.

THE POINT BEHIND THE NEEDLE

What in the world made the ancient Chinese figure out that sticking needles into the body could have a positive effect on a person's health and well-being? The idea behind it is that the body contains vital life energy (called *qi* and pronounced "chee") that runs along special invisible pathways called *meridians.* You can think of the meridians as freeways and the body's energy as the traffic that is constantly on its way from one place to the next. These freeways run up and down the arms, legs, torso, and head and also service the internal organs. In fact, each freeway is paired with a specific organ. But sometimes the traffic gets jammed and can no longer run freely. These traffic jams, or energy blockages, are believed to be the cause of disease and pain.

Luckily, the meridians flow quite near the surface of the skin in various areas, and those are the areas that are manipulated in both acupuncture and acupressure. These "acupoints" are either manipulated with the fingers or other instruments (in acupressure) or are stimulated with needles and/or electrical currents (in acupuncture). This is supposed to release the energy blockages, thus restoring and rebalancing the *qi.* Then vital functions can return to normal, the body can heal itself, and your pain or disease should go away.

Although science can't explain why acupuncture might work, it has been found to stimulate both the immune and circulatory systems. It also triggers the release of endorphins, which fight pain and depression.

WHAT GOES ON IN AN ACUPUNCTURE SESSION?

Your first visit to an acupuncturist may surprise you, for he or she will probably spend a lot of time interviewing you. The acupuncturist will not only ask you about your symptoms, how much pain you're experiencing, and your medical history but also about your diet, bowel habits, how well you sleep, and so on. The examination will extend beyond your back to include your tongue, eyes, fingernails, and skin, and the acupuncturist might take your pulse, listen to your bowel sounds and your speaking voice, and check your breathing. What does all this have to do with your back pain? Traditional Chinese medical practitioners believe that your pain is just a symptom of something that's gone awry in your body. They want to figure out what's out of balance before treating you, which makes perfect sense to me.

When it's time to receive the treatment, the acupuncturist will ask you to lie down on a padded table and loosen some of your clothing. (You won't have to undress.) Then, depending upon the diagnosis, he or she will manipulate certain acupoints (believe it or not, there are three hundred of them) by doing one or more of the following:

- *Inserting acupuncture needles*—These very thin needles are slid into place in specific acupoints and left there for anywhere from twenty to forty minutes. Don't be surprised if needles are inserted into areas that seem to have nothing to do with your back, like the back of your knee. Remember, the goal is to unblock those backed-up energy pathways, and that may require stimulation of what seems to be nonrelated areas of the body.
- *Inserting acupuncture needles and applying a low-level electrical current*—This is the way my acupuncturist likes to work. He says that adding the electrical current makes the treatment more powerful. After he's inserted the needles and hooked them up to the machine, he turns it to a low level and asks me how it feels. If I can feel a slight vibration of the nerve that's right next to each needle, that's good. If I don't feel much, he turns it up; if it's annoying or painful at all, he

turns it down. Sometimes he'll come into the room in the middle of the session and see if it's okay to turn up the machine a little. But it's always up to me.

- *Burning herbs (moxibustion)*—Sometimes an herb called mugwort (or *moxa* in Chinese) is burned over the acupuncture points to stimulate them. No, it doesn't burn your skin, it just heats it a little.
- *Cupping*—A suction-cup effect is produced when little glass cups are warmed and set on top of the acupuncture points. They stimulate the area (like a tiny massage) as they cool.

If you're like me, you might not notice a difference in the way your back feels until you've had five or six acupuncture sessions. But I found that once it began to "take," the effects of acupuncture seemed to last for up to several weeks. Now I go once a month to my acupuncturist and find that that's enough.

THE DIFFERENCE BETWEEN 'PUNCTURE AND 'PRESSURE

Acupressure is a lot like acupuncture in that it involves the stimulation of the acupoints to break up the energy blockages and to restore the normal flow of *qi.* The difference is that no needles (or electrodes) are used. The Japanese name for acupressure is *shiatsu,* and it's a very popular method of massage throughout the world. By applying pressure with the thumbs, fingers, palms of the hands, elbows, or various tools (wooden rollers, for example), the acupressurist restores energy balance and even transmits some of his or her own energy to the patient.

Done on a padded table or on a mat on the floor (for greater resistance), acupressure can be used as a warm-up before an acupuncture session, can be performed in conjunction with other kinds of massage and stretching, or can simply be done by itself. There are all kinds of techniques that the acupressurist might use—digging, kneading, plucking, pushing, vibrating, joint manipulation, even walking on your back! My acupressurist often places both of her thumbs on either side of my spine and moves them in little circles. Then she moves down an inch and repeats the motion, working her way all the way down my back. It's relaxing and stimulating at the same time and, for me, a real back pain reliever. Why does it work? Nobody is quite sure, but theory has it that the application of pressure and stimulation helps your body pump out extra endorphins (natural pain relievers), which can then trigger the release of natural anti-inflammatories. And, like all massage, acupressure stimulates the flow of blood and lymph, bringing fresh supplies of nutrients to your tissues while whisking away the wastes.

FINDING A PRACTITIONER

You can find a good practitioner of either acupuncture or acupressure at the same source: National Certification Commission for Acupuncture and Oriental Medicine (NCCAOM), 11 Canal Center Plaza, Suite 330, Alexandria, VA 22314; phone: (703) 548-9004; Web site: www.nccaom.org. The NCCAOM is the main certifying organization for acupuncturists, and with a member list of some nine thousand certified practitioners, one is bound to be located in your area.

Since acupressure (shiatsu) is practiced by a great many massage therapists, you may also be able to find an acupressurist by contacting the American Massage Therapy Association, 820 Davis Street, Suite 100, Evanston, IL 60201; phone: (847) 864-0123; E-mail: info@inet.amtamassage.org; Web site: ww.amtamassage.org.

Finally, don't overlook your doctor, chiropractor, and/or physical therapist as good referral sources for acupressure or acupuncture practitioners.

15

Stamp Out Pain with Reflexology

Can pressing on the soles of your feet relieve the aches and pains in your back? Reflexologists say that it can. By exerting pressure on specific areas on your feet, hands, or outer ears, reflexologists claim that they can relieve tension, improve circulation, stimulate nerves, and help normalize organ and gland function. Sound far-fetched? It did to me, too. Yet in China the results of over three hundred studies, covering a total of eighteen thousand individual cases and sixty-four different illnesses, showed that using reflexology helped patients improve 95 percent of the time! Reflexology has advocates in other parts of the world, too. In Denmark and Japan, many large corporations pick up the tab for reflexology under their health plans because they've found that employees who see reflexologists take fewer sick leave days.

HOW DOES REFLEXOLOGY WORK?

An ancient healing art (it dates back to the Egyptians in 2300 B.C.), reflexology is based on the idea that there are reflex areas or zones on the feet and hands that are linked to all the organs, glands, and systems of the body through the nerves. Ten "reflex-energy" zones run lengthwise through the body, each originating in one of the toes and running up the body to the top of the head, then down the arm to the finger that corresponds to that toe. On the soles of the feet, the reflex-energy zones run from each toe, straight down to the heel. The sole is also divided horizontally into four zones that correspond to major areas of the body. For example, the toes correspond to the head and neck region, the ball of the foot to the chest region, the arch of the foot to the upper and mid-abdominal region, and the heel to the lower abdominal and pelvic regions. And there are a few zones on the top side of the foot, too. All of the organs, glands, bones, and other body parts are precisely "mapped out" to correlate to one or more of these zones. The manipulation of these areas, using special thumb, finger, and hand techniques, is supposed to promote relaxation and enhance wellness, especially in the corresponding area.

REFLEXOLOGY VERSUS MASSAGE

Reflexology has a lot of the same benefits as massage. It stimulates nerve pathways and relaxes the muscles, improves blood circulation, and helps increase circulation of the lymph, whisking away some of the irritating and pain-producing by-products of metabolism. But it's also very different from massage. Massage can involve the whole body, is usually done with both hands performing rubbing and squeezing actions, works through stimulation of the muscles, and aims to improve function of the body parts that are actually touched. Reflexology, however, involves just the feet and hands and sometimes the ears, is performed mostly with the thumb and fingers, works through the stimulation of the nervous system, and aims to improve the function of *all* organs, glands, and body systems.

WHAT GOES ON IN A REFLEXOLOGY SESSION?

When the reflexologist treats you for back pain, she will stimulate all of the major reflex areas on your foot, then pay particular attention to the areas that correlate to your back. The area of the foot dedicated to the back runs straight down the big-toe side of the arch, all the way from the big toe to the heel. The inner edge of the big toe governs the cervical vertebrae (neck); the area where the big toe meets the foot governs the shoulders; the inside of the ball of the foot corresponds to the upper back; the area halfway down the foot corresponds to the waistline; and the heel area governs the lower back. There's also a spot on the outer ankle bone that corresponds to the sciatic nerve. The reflexologist will "walk the spine," which means she will work all of these areas one by one, from toe to heel.

What surprised me most when I had my first reflexology treatment was that the reflex areas aren't just on the sole of the foot, but also on the top and side of the foot, the outside of the heel, and even on the ankle! The practitioner massaged my feet a lot and rotated my ankles to loosen them up, then started in on the special thumb and finger techniques I'd been reading about. It felt like she was drawing very definite lines on the sole of my foot and up and down the insides of my toes with the side of her fingernail. Actually, she wasn't using her fingernail; it was the side of her thumb bone. But it was such a well-defined, almost sharp pressure that I was a little uncomfortable at times. She lightened up a bit but told me that it was okay if it hurt a little—it's a good hurt. So some of it felt good, some of it was a little uncomfortable, but the end result was as wonderfully relaxing as a full-body massage. When I rolled off that table after forty-five minutes, I felt like I'd had a glass of wine and an hour-long nap on the deck of an elegant cruise ship! And my feet felt relaxed, stimulated, and even a little tingly for the next twenty-four hours.

Does reflexology really work for back pain? At the moment, there's no proof that it does. But if your back pain is related to muscle tension or stress, the delicious, all-over relaxation that reflexology brings can only help.

FINDING A PRACTITIONER

To find a good reflexologist, contact the Reflexology Association of America, 4012 Rainbow Boulevard, Suite K, Box 585, Las Vegas, NV 89103-2059; phone: (702) 871-9522; Web site: www.reflexology-usa.org.

16

A Painful Way to Relieve Pain—Rolfing

The basic idea behind Rolfing is that misalignment of the body equals pain. Sound familiar? Chiropractors have been saying as much for a hundred years. The difference is that chiropractors adjust your spine to correct misalignments, while Rolfing practitioners adjust your muscles. They do this by stretching and manipulating the *fascia,* a thin, elastic membrane that's wrapped around every muscle, organ, bone, nerve, and blood vessel in your body.

A biochemist named Ida P. Rolf developed this system of bodywork in the late 1950s. She had just recovered from a respiratory problem with the help of a doctor of osteopathy, a physician who focuses on hands-on manipulation to restore balance to one's out-of-whack body alignment. Even though she was supposed to be treated for her lung ailment, the doctor treated her for body misalignment! Amazingly, it worked, setting Dr. Rolf on a path to devise her own approach to healing, based on the idea that, if your body alignment is out of line, your mental, emotional, and physical health will be out of line, as well.

When your body is misaligned, Dr. Rolf theorized, at least some of your muscles are stuck carrying an extra load. They become stressed and overly tight and start to pull the body even further out of balance. The fascia, the thin connective tissue that covers your muscles, tightens up, so muscles can't move back to their proper place by themselves. It becomes painful and difficult to move, which increases your emotional and mental stress. It's also hard to concentrate, so your ability to think clearly diminishes.

To release the fascia tightness and to "restructure" your body, the Rolfing practitioner will press really hard on various points, using fingers, knuckles, or elbows. This is done to stretch the fascia, so the muscles and other tissues can be released. No oils or lotions will be used so the practitioner can maintain good contact with your muscles. You may also be given some special breathing techniques to help release buried emotions that are causing excessive tension.

Does Rolfing work for back pain? Many people think so. One theory of back pain is that the joints in the spine become restricted or fixed—they don't want to move. And when you do move, your back "goes out." Rolfing addresses the cause of the restriction by stretching the fascia and releasing the muscles and tissues, which helps restore joint movement.

Rolfing can do other things for your back, too. It can speed the healing of back injuries by improving circulation in and around the painful area, restoring motion to the joints of the back and relieving the muscle pain arising from favoring the injured part. Rolfing can also help you learn how to adopt correct posture and to identify and eliminate bad habits that lead to more back pain—like slouching, sitting incorrectly, rolling the ankles inward, and so on.

One thing just about everybody will tell you about Rolfing is that it hurts. (Think of someone digging into your back as hard as they can with their elbows!) But, for some people, it's the best way to loosen up their back muscles and relieve pain. You may get similar results with a kind of bodywork called myofascial release, which involves the stretching and manipulation of the fascia, but this is done in a gentler way.

FINDING A PRACTITIONER

If you'd like to find a Rolfing practitioner or find out more about this kind of bodywork, contact The Rolf Institute, 205 Canyon Boulevard, Boulder, CO 80302; phone: 1-800-530-8875; Web site: www.rolf.org; or the American Massage Therapy Association, 830 Davis Street, Suite 100, Evanston, IL 60201; phone: (847) 864-0123; Web site: www.amtamassage.org.

17

Relieve Pain and Other Conditions with Herbs

Taking herbs for your back pain is sort of like taking an aspirin for a broken leg. It's certainly not going to cure you because it doesn't attack the true source of the problem. It may, however, be a nice adjunct to other treatments. First you need to address the issues of poor posture, muscle tension, conditions such as arthritis and nerve compression, incorrect lifting, overuse of shoulder purses or high heels, overly contracted muscles, and lack of exercise. But once you've got a handle on all that, you might consider herbal therapy as well.

Herbs (the leaves, seeds, stems, flowers, fruit, bark, or roots of various plants) have been used by healers for their aromatic, medicinal, or savory qualities since the beginning of time. They can be taken in many different forms—eaten raw, cooked, or dried; ground up into powder; crushed, squeezed, or steamed to remove vital ingredients that can be added to foods, supplements, drinks, or ointments; or steeped in boiling water to make tea.

Many a drug began its life as an herb. Indeed, perhaps a quarter of our modern medicines originate from plants. But a drug is more than a fancy version of an herb; it's a highly refined, stripped-down variety of one of the plant's active ingredients. Relieved of its leafy exterior and surrounding components, this active ingredient is modified, concentrated, and put into standardized form so that scientists, doctors, and patients will know the exact dosage in each pill. It's potent and pure—and, according to many, an unnatural way to knock out a disease or one of its symptoms.

Herbalists believe that in many cases an ailment can be cured or at least relieved in a more natural, less powerful way by using herbs. The active ingredients that the pharmaceutical companies turn into drugs are easier on the body but still effective (possibly even more so) when left in their natural state. And the other ingredients in the herb that surround the active ingredient can work with it to cure ills, while buffering the many side effects of a lone active ingredient that's been concentrated to unnatural levels.

This certainly sounds logical, but don't be fooled into believing that all herbs are necessarily good for you. (Think of arsenic.) Or that it's safe to take as much as you want of an herbal therapy because it's "natural." You're taking herbs because they have a medicinal effect on the body. Just as with drugs, too much medicine isn't good for you.

How do you know how much is too much? That's a tricky question since there are no set dosages of herbs. Before beginning your journey into the land of herbs, I highly recommend you find an herbalist to guide you. Self-medicating can make your problems worse or create new ones. And, since there are no set dosages for herbs and no standards of potency, it's difficult to know how much of a particular active ingredient you're actually getting. Herbs, like other plants, have a shelf life. If you buy a bottle of kava kava capsules, for example, that have been sitting on the shelf for five minutes, they're probably going to be more potent than an identical brand that has been sitting on the shelf for six months. And even if there is a freshness date on the bottle, you don't know the speed in which the herb was rushed from the field to the manufacturing plant, the effectiveness of the extraction methods, or the efficiency of the seal on the jar, and so on. Consult your herbalist for recommended dosages, but let your body tell you when a dosage "feels" correct.

A FEW QUICK DEFINITIONS

Herbalists aren't as bad as medical doctors when it comes to confusing you with big words, but they do have a few they toss around. You'll hear them speak about:

- *Extracts*—the liquefied or powdered form of a key ingredient from an herb
- *Infusions*—made by steeping an herb in boiling water so one or more key ingredients are released into the water
- *Liniments*—an herbal extract meant to be applied to the skin
- *Lozenges*—a pill made from a powdered herb or herbal oil
- *Oils*—an essential oil extracted from an herb and used for massage or aromatherapy
- *Ointments*—an herb or tincture mixed with Vaseline, wax, or another substance and applied to the skin
- *Tinctures*—made by steeping an herb in alcohol

SOOTHING HERBS FOR PAIN

There are no herbs that can permanently eliminate back pain, but several can help:

- *Meadowsweet*—A sweet, fragrant herb that makes a delightful tea, meadowsweet contains salicylic acid, an aspirin-like compound that can help ease back pain.
- *Mustard*—Taken internally or made into plasters or liniment, mustard (either the black or white variety) increases the circulation and helps ease painful backaches.

- *Stinging nettle*—Although touching the live plant is something like suffering an insect bite, an ingredient in stinging nettles can help ease inflammation. It's available as an extract (to be mixed in juice or water) or in capsule form.
- *Turmeric*—One of the fragrant ingredients in curry powder, turmeric is a natural anti-inflammatory that can help ease the pain and stiffness associated with backaches. It's also available in capsule form.

HERBS FOR ANXIETY

Many people with back pain become anxious, wondering if the pain will ever go away and desperate to get back to normal living. Here are some herbs that may help relieve that anxiety:

- *Chamomile*—A very popular herb, chamomile has gentle relaxing and sedative properties. It's often used in tea form.
- *Hops*—Known to the scientific community as *humulus lupulus,* hops help you relax. Often suggested for tension and anxiety, they are taken as an infusion or a tincture. *Caution: Hops should not be used if you're depressed, for they can worsen the problem.*
- *Lady's slipper*—Used by certain Native American groups for pain and other ailments, lady's slipper helps soothe anxiety and relieve muscle cramps. *Caution: Headaches and other problems can arise if you take large doses.*
- *Valerian*—The roots of this herb (which smells something like a stinky gym sock) are ground into powder and made into tablets or capsules. Taking a few of these at bedtime can act as a mild sedative that soothes pain, eases muscle tension, and promotes sleep. You can take as an extract (mixed with juice or water) or in capsule form. *Caution: Taking valerian*

for a long time, or taking large doses, can lead to headaches and other problems.

- *Vervain*—This herb is known for its ability to strengthen the nervous system while easing anxiety and tension. *Caution: Pregnant women and women intending to become pregnant should not take this herb.*
- *Wood betony*—Used by French herbalists for liver and gallbladder ailments, wood betony is known for its ability to calm the nervous system, relieving stress and anxiety.

HERBS TO LIFT DEPRESSION

These and other herbs may be useful in easing depression:

- *Borage*—Since ancient times, this herb has been used to lift the spirits. *Caution: Too much of a good thing, even borage, can be harmful. Take sparingly.*
- *Damiana*—Along with its ability to help lift depression, it may restore energy to the lethargic. *Caution: Excess consumption of damiana can cause headaches and other side effects.*
- *Lemon balm*—Long touted as a way to "make the sad heart merry," lemon balm was often mixed into drinks in medieval times in order to instill good cheer and courage. Aromatherapists and massage therapists often use lemon balm oil in their treatments.
- *St. John's wort*—Sometimes referred to as "nature's Prozac," St. John's wort is a mild tranquilizer, muscle relaxant, and treatment for insomnia. It can be taken as an extract (mixed in juice or water) or in capsule form.
- *Skullcap*—Depression, anxiety, insomnia, and migraines are some of the ailments that can be soothed by skullcap. In days past it was called "mad dog weed" and was used to treat

rabies. *Caution: Small doses of this herb are best, for large amounts can cause dizziness and other side effects.*

SEVERAL WAYS TO BENEFIT FROM HERBS

You don't have to eat or drink the active ingredients in herbs in order to benefit from them, for there are several other ways to enjoy their benefits.

Essential Oils

You can inhale the healing essence of herbs. A treatment called *aromatherapy* uses the volatile oils in herbs to link the healing essence of the herbs to the body's powerful senses of touch and smell. Nerves involved in the sense of smell are linked to areas of the brain that control emotions. This means that the aromas of these scented oils (called essential oils) can help call forth certain emotional responses that help to heal the mind and the body.

There are lots of essential oils that might be useful in treating back pain, including:

- *Chamomile* to ease tension
- *Geranium* to promote relaxation
- *Lavender,* an excellent relaxant and sleep aid
- *Neroli* to ease tension and anxiety and to promote sleep
- *Oil of wintergreen,* an anti-inflammatory and analgesic (pain reliever) that eases back pain, especially sciatica (inflammation of the sciatic nerve that runs from the lower spine down the back of the thigh)
- *St. John's wort* to help ease spinal pain
- *Sandalwood* to ease tension and anxiety

Essential oils are very strong, so they should never be applied in their undiluted form to the skin. Instead, a few drops should be added to a carrier oil (a mild, nonirritating oil like soybean or linseed). A good ratio is two drops of essential oil to one teaspoon of the carrier oil.

Plasters

Here's a stimulating way to ease your back pain—a good old-fashioned mustard plaster! You can make it with the prepared mustard powder that's probably sitting on your spice shelf. Put about two tablespoons of mustard powder in a bowl, add an equal amount of cold water, and mix until it forms a paste. Spread the paste on a cloth and top with one layer of gauze (to keep the paste in place). Then apply to the painful area of your back. At first it will seem cool, but soon it will begin to "heat up." Don't leave the mustard plaster on for more than ten minutes because it can be too irritating to the skin.

Poultices

Another blissful alternative is a poultice made from the dried, whole versions of chamomile, lavender, or geranium. You can make an infusion by placing the herbs in boiling water, allowing them to steep for a few minutes, and straining them from the liquid. Wrap the strained herbs in thin gauze and apply to your back. Try to keep the poultice as hot as possible, without burning your skin. (If you place a hot-water bottle on top of the poultice, it will help keep it hot longer.)

THE JOY OF HERBS

Among the greatest joys of using herbs are the sheer sensual pleasures they provide. Their taste, their aroma, and the feeling of herbal essences against our skin are delights that, in and of themselves, are healing and worthwhile experiences.

18

Homeopathy: The Minimal Dose Approach

Suppose you went to a doctor complaining about your back and were told that you need to take ant crud. That's right, you had to swallow *ant crud.* Would that be enough to make you jump up and run right out of there? It might be—unless the doctor was a homeopath and could explain to you that "ant crud" is just the nickname for the homeopathic remedy called *antimonium crudum,* and that it's sometimes used to treat arthritis of the spine. Bizarre names may not be the only thing you find strange about homeopathy, but if you give it a chance, you just might find it's got a lot to offer.

In a sense, homeopathy is a system of treating disease based on the idea that if you give a person a tiny dose of whatever it is that's ailing them, their bodies will come back stronger and fight off the disease more effectively.

The roots of homeopathy stretch back to the late 1700s. Western medicine was an iffy proposition back then, when disease was rampant and there were no modern antibiotics or other wonder drugs. Bloodletting, purging, and blistering were common practices, and the idea that doctors should wash their hands in between visiting patients was too silly to even think about. Surgical techniques were primitive, and success rates were alarmingly low. Many people were absolutely terrified of doctors, and with good reason, since their "cures" were often much worse than the disease itself.

Dr. Samuel Hahnemann was one of those Western physicians who wondered if there wasn't a better way to treat patients. One day he happened to read about the use of a certain medicine to treat malaria. He thought the information was incorrect, so he decided to take the medicine himself and see what happened. In other words, he volunteered to be his own guinea pig. To his great surprise, this cure for malaria ended up giving him the *symptoms* of malaria. But why would a medicine that cured a disease give the symptoms of that disease to a healthy person?

This little experiment prompted Dr. Hahnemann to begin an exhaustive study of medicines, from which he eventually concluded that if a substance caused mild symptoms of a certain disease in a healthy person, it could be used to cure someone who actually had that ailment. Little by little he tested various medicines and other substances, and in 1796, he published the results. His called his new system *homeopathy,* which means "same suffering."

LIKE CURES LIKE

The basic idea behind homeopathy is that like cures like. If you have Disease X, you treat it with a medicine that causes gentle symptoms of Disease X in a healthy person. It works something like a vaccine, which gives a healthy person a little piece of a disease in order to help build an immunity to it.

To formulate a remedy for whatever's ailing you, the homeopath will need to find out all about your symptoms: when they began, how they hurt, when they hurt, what seems to make the pain better or worse, and so on. And then the doctor will go further, looking beyond the symptoms to the essence of the problem. That's because the homeopath believes that your symptoms are not the real problem. Instead, they're an indication that your body is struggling with deeper physical, emotional, or mental problems. So don't be surprised if you're asked what you like to eat, what you dream about, how well you sleep, what was happening in your work/emotional/family life before your symptoms began, whether you like hot or cold weather, how you respond to stress, how you're doing at work, and so on. You'll also be asked lots of questions about your pain, more than a traditional Western physician would be likely to ask: Exactly how does the pain feel (for example, dull or sharp, sudden or achy)? When does it hurt—in the morning, noon, evening, or at night? During one season more than at others? Does it hurt more when you're upset? What makes it feel better?

Eventually, these questions (plus the physical examination) should lead the doctor to the heart of the matter, that is, to what's bugging your mind, body, and/or spirit. That's what gets treated—not necessarily the pain you're feeling right now, but the essential problem. It's treated with what's called a *constitutional remedy.* You'll be given the one remedy—chosen from among some two thousand available—that most closely mirrors the essential you, your symptoms, likes and dislikes, fear and joys, behavior, and personality.

The prescribed remedy may be in pill, tablet, powder, granule, or liquid form. The name of each remedy will be followed by a number, such as "oxalic acid 30" or "Rhus tox 6." The number refers to how diluted the remedy is. The higher the number, the more diluted—which means less of the active ingredient. But this is good, because in homeopathic theory, the smaller the dose the better.

SOME COMMON BACK PAIN REMEDIES

Although your particular remedy may be different, some of the most commonly prescribed homeopathic remedies for back pain include:

- Acetic acid for back pain that eases only when you lie on your stomach
- Aconite (*aconitum napellus*) for backs and necks that are stiff and painful
- Aesulus (*aesculus hippocastanum*) for a dull ache that resides in the lower back
- Calc fluor (*calcarea fluroica*) for a strained lower back or burning pain in the lower back
- Hydrastis (*hydrastis canadensis*) for stiff, dull pain in the lower back when help is needed to get out of a chair
- Kali carb (*kali carbonicum*) for sudden sharp pains in the lower back and shooting pains in the back and the backs of thighs
- Oxalic acid for pain between the shoulders, radiating down the arms
- Rhus tox (*rhus toxicodendron*) for pain when you get up from a reclining position
- Ruta (*ruta graveolens*) for pain in the lower back before you get up in the morning

Notice how specific the indications for the remedies are. You don't just grab any convenient pain remedy off the shelf; you look for the one that most closely matches your constitutional makeup and the essence of your ailment.

Remember, these are just examples. Your homeopathic physician may come up with a completely different remedy or combination of remedies for you.

DUELING DOCTORS

Homeopathic remedies are made from plants, minerals, and even animals. That's not surprising, for Western doctors look to the same sources for medicines. But Western doctors like to make their medicines as strong as possible, while homeopathic physicians want their treatments to be what we would call weak. Homeopathy believes that it only takes a gentle push to set the body on a healing path, so its remedies are very mild. Indeed, each one is diluted and then diluted again in liquid, until there's only a tiny part of the original substance left—maybe only one part per million.

The number of homeopathic remedies you are given, the order, and the timing depend upon what type of homeopathic physician you see. Classical homeopaths only prescribe one remedy at a time and give an absolutely minimal dose. They feel that if it starts to work within a few days or a week, great. If not, they'll try another. Modern homeopathic physicians, on the other hand, often prefer to prescribe several remedies at once.

Homeopathic medicines should always be taken with a "clean mouth," which means it's been at least ten minutes since you've had anything to eat or drink or since you've used toothpaste. Then, if your remedy is in pill form, you should either chew it or place it under your tongue to dissolve—don't wash it down with water. Powdered forms should be poured directly onto the tongue.

Homeopathic remedies are considered to be very mild. They do, however, have one side effect: You may feel worse before you feel better when taking them. That's because they often "rev up" your symptoms in order to strengthen the body's healing processes.

DOES HOMEOPATHY WORK?

Although there is no scientific proof that homeopathy works, millions of people swear by it. In fact, Britain's Queen Elizabeth has a homeopathic physician and her mother, the "Queen Mum," is a patron of the British Homeopathic Association. (She must be doing something right because she turned 100 this year!) And since there appear to be no long-lasting side effects, it's probably worth a try, if you're so inclined.

FINDING A PRACTITIONER

These days it's possible to purchase homeopathic remedies in most drugstores and supermarkets, but my advice is to see a homeopathic physician, since diagnosis and treatment are so complex and individualized. You can find one by contacting the National Center for Homeopathy, 801 North Fairfax Street, Suite 306, Alexandria, VA 22314; phone: (703) 548-7790; Web site: www.homeopathic.org.

19

Balance the Body with Ayurvedic Healing

Could meditating while fixing your gaze on precious gems help ease your back pain? How about following a special diet, taking herbs, getting massaged with scented oils, or visiting a sweat lodge? Those who believe in Ayurvedic healing (and I count myself among them) will tell you that it can make a positive difference.

A TWO-PRONGED APPROACH TO HEALING DISEASE

Ayurveda is an ancient approach to healthy living that originated in India thousands of years ago. According to Ayurvedic thought, disease comes from two sources: (1) an imbalance in the body's elements and the flow of energy (*prana*) and (2) bad karma (that is, psychological or spiritual troubles). Usually, it's the result of a combination of the two. In other words, your back pain might be a result of a combination of imbalances in your body's constitution and that long-simmering feud you've been having with your sister. For the former, treatment includes bodywork (massage), diet, herbs, and yoga. For the latter, meditation, prayer, mantras, and the use of gems may be helpful. In most cases, the disease will need to be treated both ways, soothing not just the body, but the mind, soul, and spirit as well.

DIAGNOSIS: DETRIMENTAL DOSHA

How do your body's elements and flow of energy become disturbed? According to Ayurveda, the body is made up of the same five elements that make up the universe: earth, water, fire, air, and ether. These five substances combine within the body to form the three *doshas,* or primary life forces: *vata, pitta,* and *kapha.* It's these three life forces that produce and govern the body's functions.

- *Vata,* created from a mix of air and ether, influences respiration, circulation, the nervous system, elimination, the muscles, and movements within the body's fluids and cells.
- *Pitta,* created from fire and earth, governs metabolic processes, such as digestion, and chemical reactions within the body. Pitta also "rules" the color of the skin and the temperature of the body, as well as intelligence and understanding.
- *Kapha,* created from ether and water, is responsible for growth and protection. The mucous membranes that protect our stomachs from stomach acid are under the jurisdiction of kapha, as are the fluids cushioning the brain, lubricating the joints, and moistening the skin.

Each one of us is made up of a unique combination of vata, pitta, and kapha—we're all as different as snowflakes! Some are predominantly one doshic type, others may be dual types, while still others may have fairly even mixes of the three. There is no right or wrong, no good or bad. Your dosha blend is just a unique part of your makeup. And as long as it maintains its unique balance, everything is fine. Unfortunately, it's easy to become unbalanced. Our environment, diet, exercise habits (or lack of), and other factors can cause one dosha to build up relative to the others, throwing off the internal balance. When that happens, we become ill.

DETERMINING YOUR TYPE

Ayurvedic treatment, like Western treatment, begins with a diagnosis—but instead of writing "herniated disk" on your chart, the Ayurvedic doctor will begin by determining your doshic type. That's not easy, because other things must be considered besides the three doshas. You see, there are also seven *dhatus* (tissues) to be factored into the equation. (These are muscles, fat, bone, blood, plasma, nerves, and reproductive tissues.) There is also *agni,* the energy of metabolism, and three types of *malas* (wastes): sweat, urine, and feces. As you can see, it's pretty complicated.

Doshic determination is a complex procedure that requires a skilled Ayurvedic physician. As part of the diagnostic workup, the doctor will take your pulse (in up to twelve different positions!); look at your skin, tongue, eyes, and fingernails; take urine and feces samples; smell your breath; listen to your speaking voice; and ask you many questions about your ailment, your lifestyle, and your likes and dislikes.

RESTORING THE BALANCE

Once the Ayurvedic physician identifies your imbalance, he or she can begin to ease you back to health by reducing the offending "doshic buildup" and restoring your healthy doshic balance. This can be done with a variety of techniques, including purging, enemas, sweating, fasting, massage, herbs, meditation, mantras, diet, yoga, exercise, breathing techniques, adopting or avoiding certain habits, and the use of colors, gems, and crystals.

AN AYURVEDIC TREATMENT FOR BACK PAIN

Everyone is different, so I can't tell you exactly what would be right for you, but here is an example of what an Ayurvedic physician might prescribe for back spasms:

Back spasms may be seen when there is a blockage of the energy flow in the nervous system or a wasting away of nerve tissue. In addition, the vata is generally too high. Special anti-vata herbs and/or an anti-vata diet might be required. In addition, herbs like calamus, basil, bayberry, camphor, gotu kola, guggul, turmeric, mint, and myrrh may be prescribed to clear and cleanse the nerves and brain, while restoring the flow of nerve impulses. The herbs chamomile, hops, cloves, and valerian may help relieve pain, while ashwaganda is good for easing anxiety. Certain yoga postures may be recommended, as well as meditation, visualization, and mantras to help calm and nourish the nerves. Wearing or meditating upon gems like emerald, jade, or peridot may help ease pain and improve nerve function. Gold may be suggested to strengthen your nerves, and silver to calm them. Massage with medicated sesame oil (Mahanarayan) or almond oil may help, and breathing exercises are recommended. Essential oil of sandalwood may be applied to the forehead, while oils of camphor, myrrh, frankincense, or musk can be applied to the temples to calm the nerves.

The physician may also recommend one of many classic Ayurvedic formulas or tonics made of specific herbs, such as gokshura, shatavari, or kapikacchu, or may custom blend a special one to suit your condition.

THE DIFFERENCE BETWEEN WESTERN MEDICINE AND AYURVEDA

- Western doctors zero in on the disease; Ayurveda looks for the larger imbalance.

- Western medicine wants to "zap" ailments with powerful drugs or surgery; Ayurveda aims to "balance you back to health."
- Western medicine treats us all pretty much alike; Ayurveda insists that we're all as different as fingerprints.
- Western medicine accepts a lot of side effects; Ayurveda says there should be none.

FINDING A PRACTITIONER

It's best to work with a skilled Ayurvedic doctor rather than diagnosing and treating yourself after reading a book or two. If you are interested in exploring this healing art, you can find a trained practitioner by contacting the National Institute of Ayurvedic Medicine, 584 Miltown Road, Brewster, NY 10509; phone: 1-888-246-6426; Web site: www.niam.com. A small number of Western medical doctors also practice Ayurveda.

20

Energize the Pain Away with Reiki

One of the very nice things about Reiki (which is pronounced "ray-kee") is that it doesn't hurt or taste bad. There are no injections and there's nothing to swallow; you don't have to sweat or give up anything that you like to do. All that is required is to lie back and allow the healing power of the Universe to flow in. Now, that's my kind of remedy! After huffing and puffing through hours of aerobics, dieting away those pesky love handles, stretching until I began to feel like a piece of saltwater taffy, and being Rolfed nearly to death, Reiki strikes me as absolute heaven.

THE VITAL ENERGY OF LIFE

A Japanese therapy, Reiki is based on the idea that the Universe contains—or actually is, in a sense—a life-giving energy. We all have that energy within us, and it's capable of sustaining growth, nurturing health, and healing our bodies. Unfortunately, that energy sometimes gets blocked, and then we have trouble. (You already know this drill if you've read anything about the Eastern philosophies of health and well-being, including Chinese traditional medicine and Ayurvedic healing.)

Look at it this way. We're designed to be self-healing, kind of like computers that automatically scan themselves for viruses, then eliminate them. The Universal energy acts as our virus repair program, continually scanning the mind and body for problems and fixing them. Our internal virus repair program is continually connecting with the Universal "Web site" and downloading updates, so it's never outmoded. And our self-healing is all completely automatic; we don't have to do anything but live.

CHANNELING THE ENERGY

The Universal energy normally flows to and through us all the time. But when it becomes blocked within us, we need some help getting the "juice" flowing again. Reiki practitioners help by serving as conduits or channels for the energy. The practitioner scans your body with his or her hands and can feel where the energy is blocked. Then, while you're fully clothed and relaxing, the practitioner puts his or her hands gently on these areas of your body. (Actually, the hands don't even have to come into contact with your body; they can hover about two inches above it.) The hands are placed palms down, either end to end or side by side. Twelve different areas of the body can be used, and the hands usually remain in place for about five minutes. The Universal energy flows through the practitioner into your body, clearing blocked energy channels and healing you. Since Universal energy has biologic properties, it automatically knows which part of you needs to be healed.

WHAT REIKI MAY DO FOR YOU

Reiki is used to relieve pain, lessen stress, and reduce inflammation by healing the cause of imbalances in the body and restoring the flow of energy. It's designed to promote healing, maintain wellness, and prevent illness. Reiki has been used to treat a whole slew of disorders including heart problems, insomnia, high blood pressure, digestive problems, back pain, psoriasis, migraine headaches, asthma, allergies, arthritis, and whiplash.

When you receive Reiki, you feel warmth, perhaps a tingling sensation and (after a few minutes) a very deep relaxation. I've received several Reiki treatments, and each time I've walked away with greatly diminished back pain, plus the feeling that I was somehow more complete, more a part of the world around me. My practitioner rarely does Reiki all by itself; she likes to use it in combination with massage, acupressure, reflexology, and aromatherapy. She tells me that she often performs Reiki during a bodywork session but that the client doesn't even know it. "You really don't have to stop and hold your hands over someone," she says. "You simply concentrate, bring the new energy in, and release the stagnant energy."

Reiki can be performed over and over, since there's no shortage of Universal energy and no chance of overdosing. You can even learn to perform Reiki on yourself once you've become "attuned."

FINDING A PRACTITIONER

You can find a Reiki practitioner or learn the art yourself by contacting the International Center for Reiki Training, 21421 Hilltop Street, Unit #28, Southfield, MI 48034; phone: 1-800-332-8112; Web site: www.reiki.org.

21

Release the "Morphine Within" with DLPA

Did you know that your body produces its very own brand of painkillers? And that some of those painkillers are even stronger than morphine—perhaps five hundred times stronger? These powerful painkillers are called *endorphins,* which stands for endogenous morphine, or morphine that's made from within. They're part of your body's natural, built-in pain control system.

Endorphins are the strongest painkillers in existence. When pain researchers put them to the test in experiments with animals and humans, they found that one variety, called *beta-endorphin,* was eighteen to fifty times more effective than morphine, our most powerful manufactured painkiller. Another kind of endorphin, *dynorphin,* was more than five hundred times stronger than morphine in some biological tests! And these substances are happily residing in your body, at this very minute, ready to block your pain.

HOW DO ENDORPHINS BLOCK PAIN?

To understand the action of the endorphins, you first have to know how the pain message is carried to the brain. Suppose you touch a hot stove with your finger. The neurons (nerve cells) in your fingertip release neurotransmitters, chemical messengers that help carry the message to your brain that your body is being damaged. The neurotransmitters hop across tiny spaces between one neuron and the next by binding to a special receptor site on each "new" neuron. Thus, the message is carried from neuron to neuron until it reaches your spinal cord and is rocketed to your brain. Your brain then sends its own "get finger off stove" message back to your fingertip, and you jerk your hand away from the stove before you've even figured out what's happened. This pain message to brain/action message back to body process is a wonderful thing in the case of acute pain (the kind of pain that occurs in response to something that's happening right now and needs attention). But, in the case of chronic pain, the kind of pain that goes on and on, these pain messages are not so helpful.

That's when endorphins can truly be a blessing. Naturally produced by the body, they sneak in and bind to the receptor sites in the neurons, blocking the pain message from heading up to the brain. It's sort of like Goldilocks sneaking into Baby Bear's bed. If she's already in the bed, he has nowhere to sleep. Similarly, if the endorphins bind to the neurotransmitter's receptor sites, the pain message can't get through.

The body makes endorphins, and the body destroys them. We don't want their levels to rise too high and block too much pain. We need some pain, at least enough to tell us to take our hands off those hot stoves! Without pain telling us something is wrong, we'd be constantly stubbing our toes, burning our hands, not noticing the problems in our arthritic joints, and otherwise failing to take care of ourselves.

STOCKING UP ON ENDORPHINS

Clearly, a great way to relieve pain is to make sure you've got a plentiful supply of endorphins. So, why aren't we just injecting endorphins into our painful backs and going about our business? Scientists tried that, but the endorphins were quickly broken down by enzymes in the body, so the pain relief only lasted about twenty minutes. In order to be really effective, the endorphins would have to be injected directly into your brain or spinal cord—and that, of course, is dangerous, complicated, and expensive. How about endorphins in pill form? Sorry. The digestive juices in your stomach and gastrointestinal tract would break them down before they could be of any use.

Since we can't seem to increase our endorphin supplies from without, we need something to "pump up" the endorphins we've already got, and to do it from within. And that something is a nutritional supplement called DLPA.

DLPA TO THE RESCUE

DLPA is a shorter, easier way of saying dl-phenylalanine (pronounced "dee-ell-fennel-al-a-neen"). DLPA is nothing more than a version of a simple amino acid that's found in some of the foods we eat.

Phenylalanine is a common amino acid found in our foods and in our bodies. It's called PA for short. PA comes in two forms, the "d" and the "l." You can think of the "d" form, or DPA, as the "right-handed" form, and the "l" form, or LPA, as the "left-handed" form. The two forms are mirror images of each other, like your right and left hands. DLPA is a 50/50 mixture of DPA and LPA.

DLPA can help relieve your pain in several of the following ways:

- It protects your endorphins from destruction. This allows your body to build up its supply of these natural pain relievers and makes them last longer.
- It makes it easier for endorphins and their receptors to connect, a necessary step in pain relief.

- It helps relieve depression (and depression worsens pain).
- It increases the pain-relieving effects of drugs like aspirin, acetaminophen, and ibuprofen.
- It's a natural anti-inflammatory agent.

The Endorphin Shield

DLPA can actually help increase the amount of endorphins in your blood by slowing down the action of certain "endorphin-chewing" enzymes. Shielded from their natural enemies, endorphins can flourish—increasing in number and living longer. That translates to better, longer-lasting relief from chronic pain. (DLPA doesn't work for acute pain, so don't try to cure a headache with it. It must be taken over a period of time, and it works on chronic pain only.)

The Endorphins Meet the Receptors

A breakdown product of DLPA makes it easier for endorphins and their receptors to connect and form a bond that is sort of like a lock and key. (Until endorphins connect with their receptors, they can't start to relieve your pain.) The breakdown product is called PEA, or phenylethylamine (pronounced "fennel-ethel-am-een"). PEA may also encourage the release of more endorphins.

Lessen the Depression

PEA also helps relieve depression, and anyone who's ever been depressed knows that it can make your pain even worse. Several studies have shown that depressed patients have much lower levels of PEA in their body fluids than do nondepressed patients. Lots of antidepression therapies, including drugs, work (in part) by raising PEA levels. PEA is also associated with the euphoric feeling of falling in love (!). By taking DLPA, you'll raise your PEA levels and automatically elevate your mood.

Another way DLPA fights the depression "bug" is by increasing the amount of a stimulant manufactured in the brain called norepinephrine.

Buffing Up the Bufferin

Conventional pain pills don't work for very long, and they often have to be taken several times a day. Demerol, for example, is usually taken every three to four hours, aspirin every four hours, and Percodan every six hours. But the pain-relieving effects of DLPA last approximately five days, and when taken with over-the-counter pain remedies like aspirin, they can last as long as seven days! This longer-lasting effect also occurs when DLPA is taken with acetaminophen and ibuprofen.

Fighting Inflammation

DLPA is also good at fighting inflammation. When lab animals were injected with a chemical that causes severe inflammatory reactions, DLPA was able to reduce the reactions significantly in 78 percent of the animals. Other studies have found it helpful in controlling the inflammation found in arthritis.

DLPA IS SAFE!

Even though DLPA can do all of these things, it appears to be utterly safe to take. It's long-lasting, nonaddictive, has no adverse side effects, and is nontoxic. Do I sound like an advertisement for DLPA? If so, it's only because I've found it so very helpful in keeping my neck pain at bay. My brother-in-law, a medical doctor who also believes in alternative medicine, first recommended DLPA to me. When my neck is bugging me and won't quit, I take DLPA three times a day for the next several weeks. The pain pretty much disappears and stays away (sometimes for months!) even after I've stopped taking the supplement. It makes a lot more sense to me than loading up on aspirin (or stronger drugs). Why not try buffing up your own natural resources?

Caution: People with the genetic disease called phenylketonuria (PKU) should not take DLPA because they cannot properly metabolize the amino acid. Anyone else on a phenylalanine-restricted diet should avoid DLPA, as should pregnant and lactating women, and children.

HOW TO TAKE DLPA

My brother-in-law recommends taking 375 milligrams of DLPA three times a day, with meals. If you don't get pain relief after three days of this, increase the dose to 750 milligrams. DLPA is available in vitamin and health food stores.

Of course, you should consult your doctor before self-medicating with DLPA.

22

Minimize Pain with Magnets

I resisted the use of magnets for a long time before trying them. It seemed so silly to me—as if pain were a brass pin that you could suck up with something that sticks to the refrigerator door! To tell you the truth, it was vanity that drove me to it. My husband and I had decided to do a little demonstration of the swing dancing we'd learned recently, and the forum we'd picked was my father-in-law's seventy-fifth birthday party. While Jack was whirling me around during practice one day, I snapped something in the back of my right knee. (Okay, I confess, I was wearing high heels at the time!) Anyway, I needed to get my knee back in shape in a hurry because the party was just two weeks away, and we had to get a lot more practice time under our belts.

Since magnets are just about everywhere these days (the pharmacy, the grocery store, mail-order catalogs, even department stores), it was just a matter of time until one of them caught my eye. I happened to be in the elastic bandage section of our local drugstore when I saw a knee support that contained twenty-six magnets. At that point I was so desperate I was willing to try anything, so I bought it.

Thirty minutes after I'd pulled this magnetized support over my knee, the pain had disappeared! I'm not kidding. At first I thought it was all in my head, but my knee continued to have little or no pain from that point on.

So what does all of this have to do with back pain? Well, I decided that since the magnets had worked so effectively on my knee, I'd try them on my back and neck, and I do think they've helped. I haven't had the dramatic "healing experience" that I had with my knee, but they've definitely been useful.

MAGNETIC THEORY 101

There is a certain amount of science behind the idea that magnets can quell your pain. You might remember from elementary school that magnets generate a magnetic field and have a positive pole and a negative pole. The effect of the magnetic field on the body hasn't yet been proven, but many experts think that the negative pole can help normalize body functions and exert a calming effect. The magnetic field may also interrupt the flow of pain signals to the brain, cause the release of endorphins (our old friend, the pain-fighter), and increase circulation in the painful area. Magnetic therapy is currently used to help speed the healing of broken bones.

DOES IT WORK?

Although research on magnetic therapy was only begun recently, there is one good study that shows that magnets can have a positive effect on back pain. Fifty patients with back pain due to post-polio syndrome were divided into two groups. One group was given magnets and told to place them on their painful areas for forty-five minutes. The other group was given inactive magnets with the same instructions. Afterward, 75 percent of those who received the real magnets had significantly less pain, compared to only 19 percent of those with the inactive magnets (whose pain only decreased a little). Those who used the real magnets reported that their pain relief lasted anywhere from a couple of hours to several months.

HOW TO USE MAGNETS FOR PAIN RELIEF

You can find magnets in lots of different forms: embedded in belts or wraps (like the one I got for my knee); put into pillows or mattress covers; in beds, bracelets, or the inner soles of shoes; or as disks that you can tape to the painful area. I suggest that you try the cheapest variety first (probably the disks or a back belt) to find out if magnetic therapy does anything for you. You certainly don't want to invest hundreds of dollars in a magnetic bed, only to find that your back still hurts!

Place the magnets directly on your skin whenever possible. The more wrapping or padding between the magnet and your painful area, the weaker the magnetic field, and the more watered-down the effects. Conversely, the greater the magnetic field, the greater the effects, so you should also pay attention to the strength of the magnet, which is listed on the package as gauss or Telsa. The magnetic field of the earth is 0.05 gauss, and a refrigerator magnet has about 60 gauss, while 10,000 gauss equal 1 Telsa. Get the strongest magnets you can find.

WARNING! MAGNETIC THERAPY IS NOT FOR EVERYBODY

If you have a pacemaker or other implanted electronic device, or if you're pregnant, check with your doctor before using magnets. Magnets should never be placed directly over an electronic implant or on the abdomen during pregnancy.

23

Learn to Relax!

We've all heard a lot about the mind-body connection: the theory that thinking certain thoughts can affect the state of your physical body. This isn't just somebody's idealistic notion; there are scores of scientific studies showing that what you think can make a huge difference in your health, for better or for worse. Never is this more true than with back pain, which is either directly caused or made much worse by stress and the way a person handles that stress.

WHY IS STRESS SO HARMFUL?

When mental or physical demands are made on you, your body rises to the occasion in the same basic way that a caveman's body responded back in prehistoric times. Your blood pressure and heart rate increase, your breath comes harder and faster, your muscles tense, and your body becomes flooded with stress hormones to give you a sudden burst of energy. These hormones (which include adrenaline, cortisol, and other high-powered natural chemicals) gave the caveman the ability to fight off an angry grizzly bear or run for his life from a band of invading tribesmen. Your stress, though, is not usually due to grizzly bears or tribesmen on the warpath. More often it's due to getting the runaround from a credit-card billing department or being cut off by a rude driver on the freeway. Yet your physical reaction is exactly the same as the caveman's. The difference is, he probably used the physical changes triggered by stress to run a mile or engage in battle. You, on the other hand, are left to stew in your own juices as you sit in your car and glare at the other driver.

Every time you go through another stressful incident, your body is flooded with powerful chemicals. Over time, this can do a lot of damage. Headaches, insomnia, stomach problems, high blood pressure, and back pain can all be rooted in too much stress, or stress that's dealt with improperly. That's why it's crucial to take some time each day to let that stress go. You can reverse many of the physiological changes brought on by stress just by learning to relax. You can consciously lower your blood pressure, reduce the level of stress hormones in your blood, decrease your heart rate, let go of muscle tension, reduce anxiety, and ease your pain by using one of several techniques that bring about the relaxation response.

THE RELAXATION RESPONSE

It's important to understand the difference between the relaxation response and just hanging around, relaxing. I'm not talking about watching TV, lying on the couch, reading, or whatever you do to relax. A true relaxation response means that the physiological functions of the body slow down markedly. In order to do this, according to Dr. Herbert Benson of Harvard Medical School, you need four things:

1. *A mental device*—You need something to focus on that will take your mind off what normally preoccupies you. You're not going to be able to relax very well if your head keeps replaying that fight you had with your husband over and over again. Mantras and relaxation tapes are good mental devices.

2. *A passive attitude*—This means that you shouldn't try too hard to relax or to do anything else when you're practicing a relaxation technique. It's not a competition, and trying to be perfect is counterproductive. Just focus on the mental device. If stray thoughts cross your mind (which they will), accept that they're there and gently bring your focus back to your mental device.
3. *A lessening of muscle tension*—Get into a comfortable position, either sitting or lying down, so your muscles don't have to work too hard to hold you up.
4. *Peace and quiet*—Find a place free from noise and distractions where you won't be interrupted. It's hard to relax when people keep barging in on you!

Once you've got the right setup, you'll be able to elicit the relaxation response whenever you wish by using techniques such as deep breathing, meditation, progressive relaxation, and biofeedback.

TECHNIQUES TO ELICIT THE RELAXATION RESPONSE

Deep Breathing

The next time you find yourself really stressed, step outside of yourself for a minute and notice how you're breathing. I'll bet you'll be taking short, shallow, quick breaths, with the in-and-out motion all in your upper chest. But just by taking a slow, deep breath that fills up your entire lungs, then slowly exhaling, you can begin to relax. Deep breathing is a big part of many relaxation and stress reduction techniques and can be used to control pain, lower blood pressure, quell panic attacks, and control negative emotions.

Done properly, deep breathing expands the rib cage and diaphragm more than the chest. You'll be able to teach yourself the right way to do deep-breathing exercises by lying on your back and placing your hand lightly on your diaphragm area, just below the center of your rib cage. Breathe in slowly to the count of five and allow your rib cage and stomach to push outward. Hold for a count of five, then slowly release for a count of five. When you're ready, take another deep breath, using the same techniques. Do five to ten breaths total, then let your breathing go back to normal. You should find yourself well on the way to total relaxation!

Meditation

For thousands of years, meditating has been an important tool for those seeking spiritual enlightenment. It's also a great way to "center" yourself, to escape from the pressures and tensions of a fast-paced world, to improve both your physical and mental health, and to ease your pain.

The mental device used in meditating can be whatever you want it to be—a sound, a phrase, the in-and-out movement of the breath, a particular color, or an object. Some people meditate on the flame of a candle or a special word that is given to them by their teachers. Whatever device you use, the process is the same.

In a quiet place where you can be alone for at least twenty minutes, sit in a comfortable position on the floor and close your eyes. You may want to sit on a mat or pillow, and many people like to sit in a cross-legged position because it's the most comfortable way to sit for long periods of time. If it hurts your back to do this, though, feel free to lean against the front of a chair or some kind of backrest. (Don't lie down because you'll probably fall asleep!)

Silently repeat to yourself the word or sound that you've chosen, slowly and rhythmically. Or, if you're focusing on your breathing instead, notice how the air flows all the way into your body, filling up every part, then is slowly released, taking away all wastes and pain. If you're using a physical object as your mental device, keep your eyes open and simply concentrate on it. As stray thoughts enter your mind, acknowledge them and let them go. Continue this process for twenty minutes, then slowly open your eyes, stretch, and ease back into your daily life.

It may be hard to concentrate on one thing for a full twenty minutes, but meditation is a way of disciplining the mind and allowing it to rest at the same time. It takes practice, but, like most things, it gets easier over time.

Progressive Relaxation

The special mental device in progressive relaxation isn't a word or phrase but the feel of your own muscles. Listening to a guide, using an audiotape, or just hearing the tape inside your own head, you'll concentrate on tightening up the muscles, ligaments, and tendons in one area (say, your head), then consciously relaxing them. Next, you'll tighten your neck muscles and slowly relax them. The tightening and relaxing progress all the way through your body, down to your toes. (Sometimes, progressive relaxation concentrates only on the relaxation part, without the tightening up.) By the time you've gone through every body part this way, you can find yourself so relaxed that all you want to do is roll over and sleep! That's where audiotapes come in handy—you can use them in bed and just drift off into dreamland once you've completed the exercise.

Biofeedback

Biofeedback is an excellent tool for teaching you how to relax and how to sustain the relaxation response. That's because it lets you know what's going on inside your body, and it shows you instantaneously how your body is responding to its environment.

You may feel like a science experiment during biofeedback sessions, but it will be worth it in terms of the new insight you'll get into how your body works and how you can control it. You'll be hooked up to a machine that monitors your heart rate, blood pressure, body temperature, muscle tension, and other functions. A beeping sound will indicate your heartbeat, and you'll see readouts of your temperature, blood pressure, respiration rate, and so on.

Once you're hooked up, you'll start to practice your relaxation techniques, and, amazingly, you'll be able to see the changes in your body. The beep for your heartbeat will sound less often, and you'll be able to watch your blood pressure and respiration rates drop. As you learn what works, you can practice and become even more proficient at controlling your bodily responses. It's great fun and very impressive!

FINDING A PRACTITIONER

You can find someone who can teach you about deep breathing, meditation, or progressive relaxation by contacting the Mind-Body Medical Institute, New England Deaconess Hospital, One Deaconess Road, Boston, MA 02215; phone: (617) 632-9525; Web site: www.mindbody.harvard.edu; or the Stress Reduction Clinic, University of Massachusetts Medical Center, Worcester, MA 01655; phone: (508) 856-2656.

You can find a biofeedback practitioner through the Association for Applied Psychophysiology and Biofeedback, 10200 West 44th Avenue, Suite 304, Wheat Ridge, CO 80023; phone: 1-800-477-8892; Web site: www.aapb.org.

24

See Yourself as Pain Free

Nearly two thousand years ago, the Roman emperor Marcus Aurelius declared that "our lives are what our thoughts make of it." His sentiments are as true today as they were back then. If you can conceive of something, you can probably find a way to achieve it. But if you just can't imagine that you can reach a certain goal, well, you probably won't.

Healers have long known about the *placebo effect,* the ability of a sugar pill or other ineffective substance to make patients feel better and even recover completely because they believed the "medicine" would work. Obviously the sugar pill didn't cure anything—it had to be the positive thoughts. In the 1970s and 1980s, scientists started to explore this connection between positive thinking and health. And they found something very interesting.

Researchers studying elderly Jewish men, for example, found that their mortality rates dipped significantly right before Passover, an important Jewish holiday. After the holiday was over, the death rate soared—almost as if it were compensating for the earlier decline—and then returned to the normal level. What was the explanation? The men were looking forward to the holiday, even willing themselves to live by sending themselves positive mental messages. But once the holiday was over, they no longer had the need or the will to live. They'd postponed death long enough, now they could pass on.

A similar study was done with elderly Chinese women and the Harvest Moon Festival, a celebration that pays special attention to older females. Once again, the death rate dropped before the holiday, then rose above normal afterward, before settling down to its typical level.

POSITIVE THINKING FOR BACK PAIN RELIEF

Okay, so thinking positively may be able to keep the Angel of Death at bay, at least for a while. But what can it do for your back pain? Scientists at the University of Tennessee Health Sciences Center looked at a group of people suffering from back pain that didn't seem to respond to any kind of treatment. They measured their endorphin levels, then gave them a placebo. But they told the patients that it was a brand-new medicine that would make them feel better. Thirty percent of the patients soon found themselves feeling better. The researchers measured the endorphin levels in these people again and found that they had risen. It was the extra endorphins that were blocking their pain, but what made the endorphin levels rise? Undoubtedly, it was the patients' positive thoughts.

SEE IT IN YOUR MIND'S EYE

To harness the power of positive thinking and put it to work relieving your back pain, you've got to use your imagination. Two techniques can help you do this: visualization and guided imagery. You can learn both from books or tapes, but it's best to find a teacher who can take you through these processes several times so you know just what to do. Then these techniques will be yours to use whenever you choose. Both techniques should be done in a quiet, restful place where you won't be disturbed. Turn the lights down low, light a candle, and play soft, relaxing music, if you like. Then do some deep breathing, meditation, yoga postures, and/or progressive relaxation for a few minutes. When you're feeling very relaxed, you're ready for visualization and/or guided imagery.

Visualization

Your instructor will ask you to visualize an image (it could be a place, a person, or an object) that has strong meaning for you and brings up particular feelings. In the case of back pain, you may be asked to think of a place where you have felt very, very relaxed and peaceful and your back was completely well. You'll imagine the scene in minute detail: where you are, what it looks like, who is with you, whatever smells you can conjure up. Then you'll be asked to recall how your back felt when you were in that place. You'll see yourself getting up and moving around with no pain—you're bending, twisting, walking, running, even jumping while your back feels absolutely fine.

Regularly visualizing yourself as healthy and well and feeling positive about yourself (and especially your back) should increase your endorphin levels, lower your stress levels, and boost your immune system.

Guided Imagery

In this process, an instructor (or a voice on a tape recording) will do the imagining for you, taking you on a verbal "trip" to a better, more relaxed, healthier place where you can dwell for a while before easing back into reality. The instructor may take you to a place where you'll "see" your pain literally melting away or you'll imagine yourself doing something physical that you don't ordinarily do—with ease. Often, guided imagery is used as a relaxation tool. Here's an example of guided imagery that's aimed at relaxing you so completely that you fall asleep:

> Imagine that you are at the top of a long flight of stairs. But these aren't ordinary stairs—they are covered with plush, cranberry-colored velvet that has very deep, soft, fluffy padding underneath. As you step onto the first step, your right foot sinks down into that plush cranberry velvet, and it feels very soft and comforting. Then your left foot steps onto the next step and sinks into the velvet, easing down into the thick, soft padding. You keep stepping, now with your right foot, sinking down, down into the velvet, now with your left foot, sinking, sinking. Keep walking, first with your right foot, then your left, and you sink each time into the soft, comfortable padding as you progress down the stairs.
>
> Now, as you near the bottom of the stairs, you notice that you are getting very sleepy, so sleepy that all you want to do is lie down and drift into a deep, comfortable sleep. You see a soft, cozy bed covered with cranberry velvet at the bottom of the stairs. It has fluffy, deliciously squishy pillows and the softest flannel sheets. You crawl into that wonderful, comfortable bed, pull the covers over yourself, sink into those pillows, and fall fast asleep.

FINDING A PRACTITIONER

If you'd like to find someone who can teach you about visualization and guided imagery, contact the Academy for Guided Imagery, P.O. Box 2070, Mill Valley, CA 94942; phone: 1-800-726-2070; Web site: www.healthy.net/agi.

25

You *Do* Have a Prayer

What if I told you there was a magic pill that could relieve your stress, ease your pain, and speed your recovery time? Not only that, it could provide you with a sense of belonging, offer comfort, help you keep your pain in perspective, and give you the feeling that the greatest doctor in the world is looking after you. Unfortunately, no such pill exists, but many people do reap these benefits from good old-fashioned prayer.

This will come as no surprise to the 76 percent of us who pray regularly, and the 79 percent of us who believe that faith in God or a Higher Power can help us heal faster and better. And researchers are beginning to agree that prayer can, indeed, be a powerful medicine.

Various studies have shown that regularly attending religious services can be good for your health. People who go to services (compared to those who don't)

- take better care of their health,
- are less likely to be hospitalized,
- are more likely to be released from the hospital sooner,
- recover faster from major surgery,
- live longer.

And a study of seniors who were hospitalized and depressed found that those who were spiritual bounced back from depression sooner.

But you don't have to belong to a religious group or go anywhere special to benefit from prayer. Prayer is an affirmation of yourself, your life, your place in the world, a Higher Power who looks after you, and the Universe itself. And that can be done anywhere, anytime. You just have to take some quiet time and look into your own soul. After all, what are we really saying when we pray? We are saying that there is an order to the Universe and a place for us within it; that someone loves and cares for us; that there is a reason to gravitate toward good and shun evil; that we have the power to do many things, but ultimately the power lies in the hands of something greater than ourselves; that we love and are loved. Knowing these things and affirming our faith in love, peace, and a Higher Power can bring a sense of peace and well-being that improves mental, emotional, physical, and spiritual health on every level.

Prayer works—and not only for those who pray but also for those who are in the prayers of others. You may be surprised to hear that researchers have uncovered scientific proof of this! One study involved patients with heart disease, half of whom were prayed for by a Christian group. None of the patients knew that they were being prayed for, and those who prayed didn't know the patients personally. The group that was prayed for had fewer complications than the group that was not prayed for. A similar study of AIDS patients showed that those who were prayed for developed fewer new illnesses, had less severe symptoms, and went to the doctor less often than those not included in the prayers.

Prayer is like a concentrated version of positive thinking plus visualization and creates thoughts that can strengthen your immune system and tip your body's biochemical balance in favor of radiant health. So pray—pray for whatever you desire and believe that it will come true. See yourself reaching your goals and enjoying them immensely! Visualize yourself as healthy, happy, pain-free, and able to do whatever catches your fancy. See your prayers coming true. You will be amazed at the results.

Afterword

Now that I've waxed euphoric over my twenty-five remedies for back pain, I thought you might want to know how they've worked on my own back and neck problems. I can honestly say that I haven't had a back attack in over a year, although my neck still bothers me sometimes. When I just can't stretch the tension out of it, I drag myself back to Dr. Dan and get him to do a little Trigger Point Therapy on my neck and shoulder muscles. That seems to be the best thing for me.

As for my overall back health, it's greatly improved in the last couple of years. The things I've done that I think have helped me most are

- improving my posture (both sitting and standing),
- going to dance class regularly (for stretching and strengthening my back muscles),
- wearing high heels only once in a while, and
- getting a good desk chair that supports my lower back.

The things I'm still working on are

- learning to sleep in more back-friendly positions,
- practicing relaxation techniques on a regular basis, and
- eating more fruits and vegetables (shouldn't everybody?).

Living with back pain can be debilitating, depressing, and infuriating. It can sideline you and suck all of the joy out of your life. *But it doesn't have to!* You can take control of your back pain, your health, and your life. Remember: Attack the mechanical problems first, since almost all back problems begin there. But don't be afraid to try some of the alternative treatments as well. Your own personal recipe for back pain relief will probably call for a little of this, a lot of that, and a smidgen of the other. Experiment—it's the only way you'll find out what works.

May yours become as strong as the back of a weight lifter, as supple as the back of a gymnast, and as pain-free as the back of a young child—preferably one who does cannonball flips off the diving board without thinking twice!

Index

E

F

G

H

T